The Complete

RENAL

DIET

COOKBOOK

20 quick and easy recipes to manage and improve kidney functions

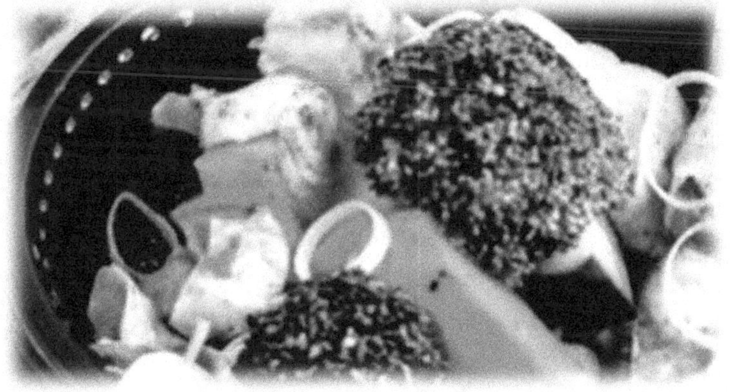

Dr. Grace Hester A.kaboo Publishing —

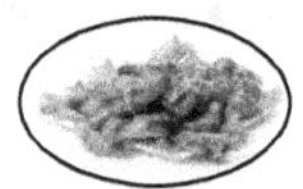 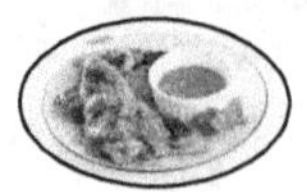 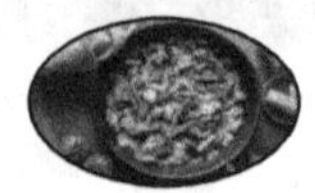

Copyright Page

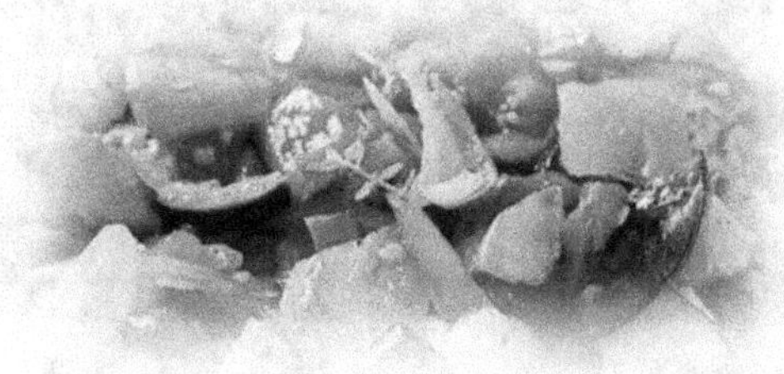

DR. GRACE HESTER

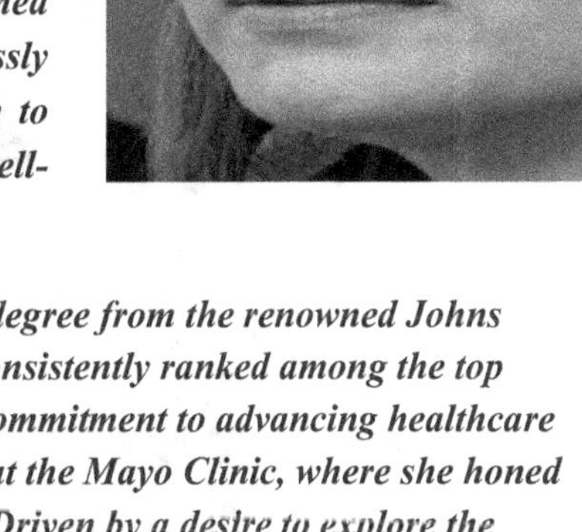

.Dr. Grace Hester stands at the intersection of health, passion, and culinary excellence. A distinguished medical professional and accomplished nutritionist, she seamlessly weaves together her expertise to create a holistic approach to well-being.

Dr. Hester earned her medical degree from the renowned Johns Hopkins School of Medicine, consistently ranked among the top medical schools globally. Her commitment to advancing healthcare led her to prestigious positions at the Mayo Clinic, where she honed her skills in internal medicine. Driven by a desire to explore the profound connection between nutrition and overall health, she furthered her education at the Culinary Institute of America.

– With a deep understanding of both medicine and nutrition, Dr. Hester embarked on a mission to inspire others to embrace a healthier lifestyle. Her culinary journey– led to the creation of a series of cookbooks that blend the art of cooking with the scienc–e of nutrition. Each recipe is a testament to her commitment to flavor, nourishment, and well-being.

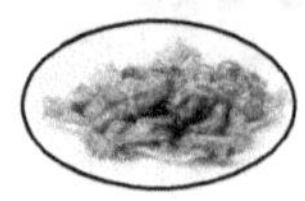 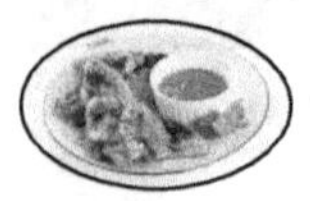 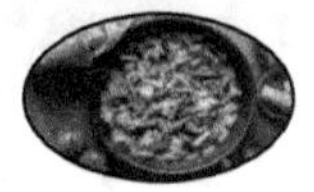

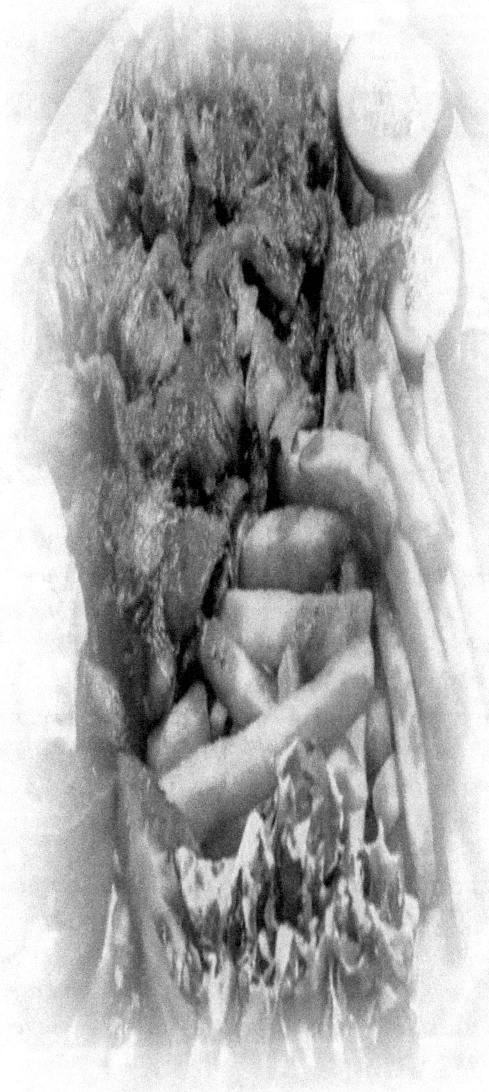

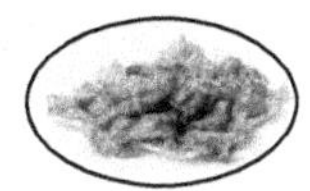 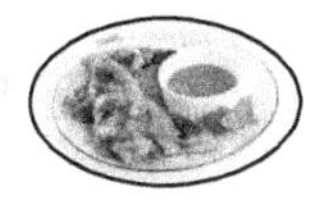 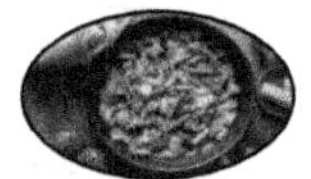

TABLE OF CONTENT

INTRODUCTION–..**9**

1. Grilled Lemon Herb Chicken..**13**

2. Herb-Roasted Salmon..**14**

3. Quinoa and Vegetable Stir-Fry.....................................**16**

4. Turkey and Vegetable Chili...**17**

5. Baked Lemon Garlic Tilapia..**19**

6. Vegetable and Lentil Soup..**20**

7. Spinach and Feta Stuffed Chicken Breast....................**22**

8. Mango Salsa Shrimp Tacos...**23**

9. Eggplant and Tomato Casserole...................................**24**

10. Lemon Dill Baked Cod...**26**

11. Vegetarian Chickpea Salad...**27**

12. Cauliflower Rice Pilaf..**29**

13. Sweet Potato and Black Bean Tacos..........................**30**

14. Turkey and Vegetable Skewers...................................**32**

15. Creamy Asparagus Risotto..**33**

16. Chicken and Vegetable Curry.....................................**35**

17. Shrimp and Broccoli Stir-Fry.......................................**37**

18. Mushroom and Spinach Stuffed Bell Peppers.............**38**

19. Lentil and Vegetable Curry Soup................................**40**

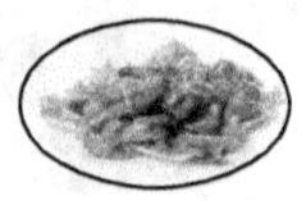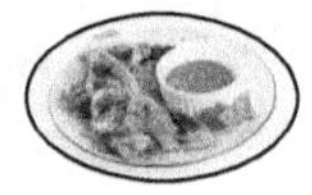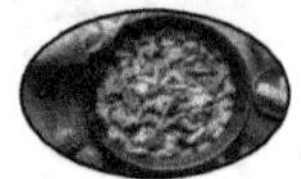

20. Tofu and Vegetable Stir-Fry...42

WE KNOW… 47

20 DAYS + MEAL PLANNER... 48

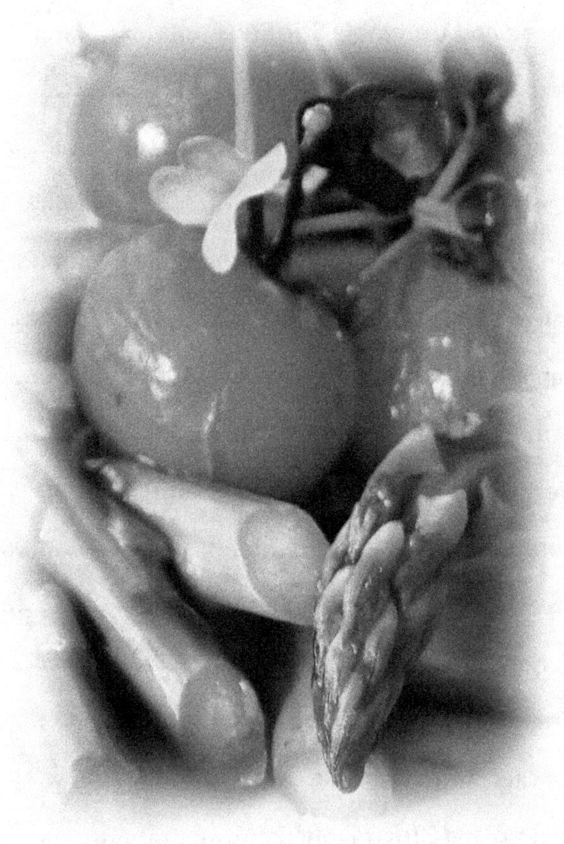

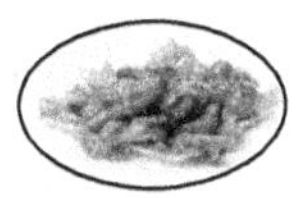 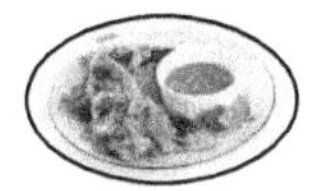 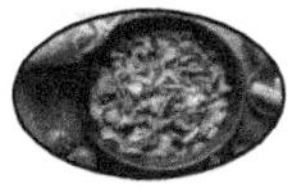

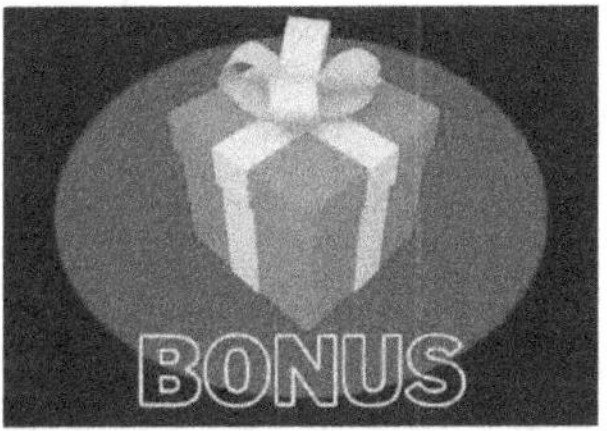

SCAN THE QR CODE TO GET YOUR FREE HOME

MADE GREEN SMOOTHIE RECIPE BOOK

Your 20 days meal planner is attached at the end of the book. Enjoy!

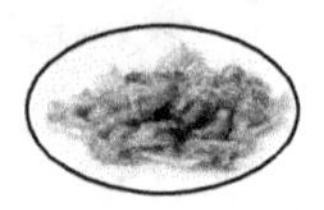 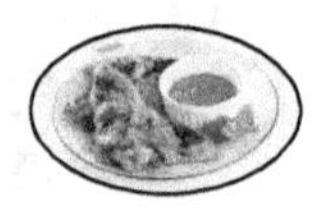 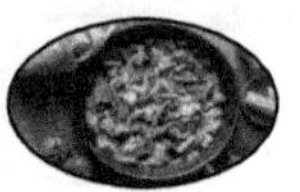

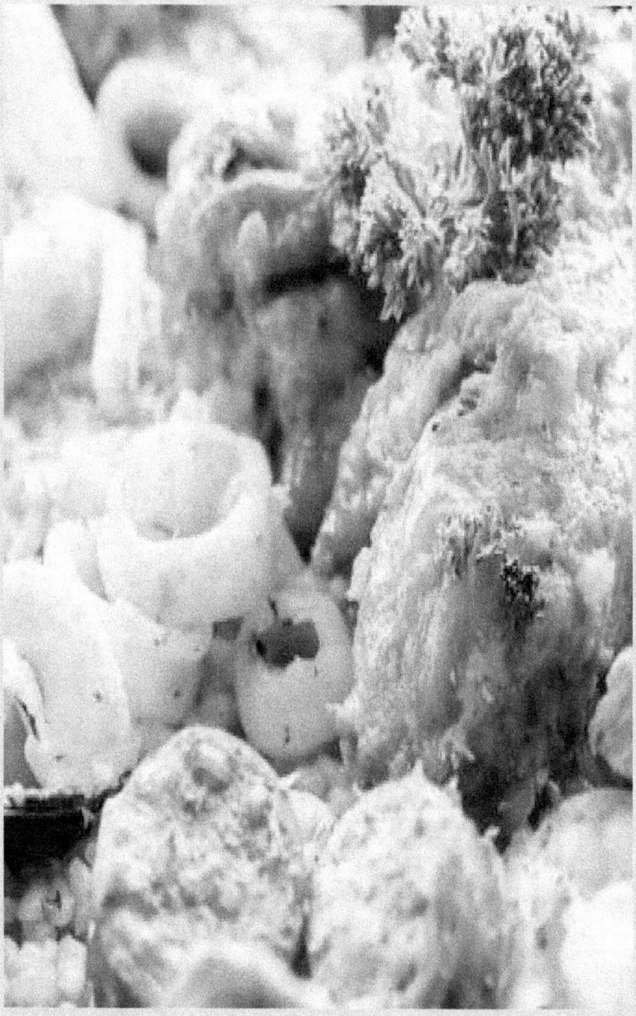

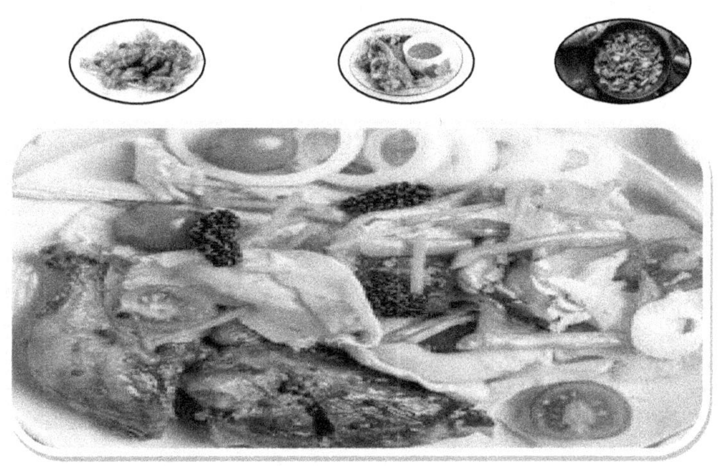

INTRODUCTION-

In the quiet corners of the culinary world, where flavor meets function and health intertwines with taste, emerges a gastronomic journey like no other. Welcome to "The Renal Rejuvenation Cookbook," a culinary expedition designed to transform your kitchen into a sanctuary of well-being.

In the enchanting realm of nutrition, where every ingredient tells a story and every recipe is a chapter, we embark on a narrative aimed at managing and reversing the tides of kidney disease. Picture a kitchen as a canvas, where the brushstrokes are strokes of vitality, and each dish is a masterpiece sculpted to nourish not only the body but the spirit.

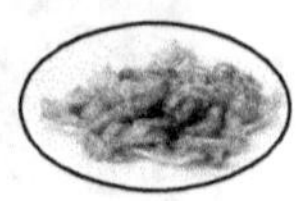 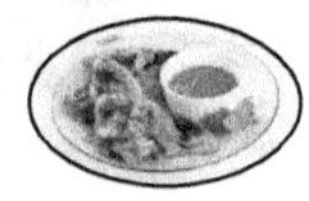 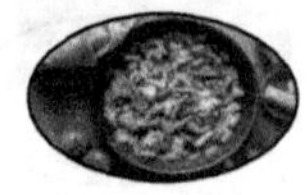

As we delve into the heart of this cookbook, we unravel the tales of Grilled Lemon Herb Chicken, where succulent chicken breasts dance with the zesty notes of lemon and a symphony of herbs. The pages turn, revealing the secrets of a creamy Asparagus Risotto, a comforting embrace of Arborio rice and tender asparagus that whispers promises of both indulgence and health.

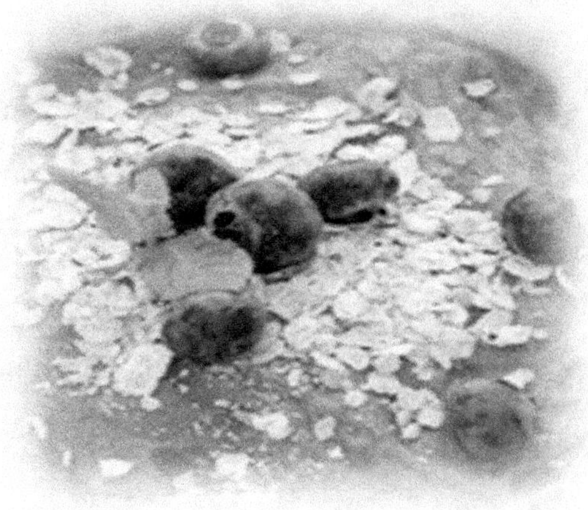

Through each recipe, we discover that the path to renal wellness need not be mundane or restrictive. It is a culinary odyssey that leads us to explore the depths of flavor in –

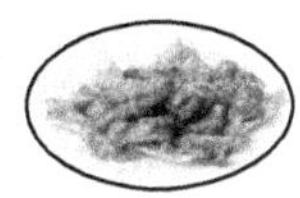 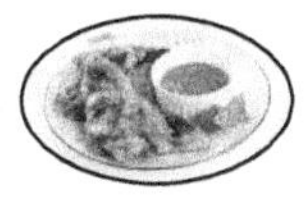 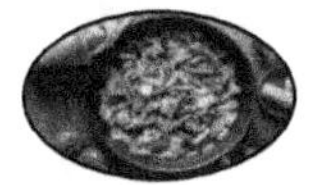

Sweet Potato and Black Bean Tacos, where the vibrant colors of nature converge on your plate, bringing joy to both the eyes and the palate.

Join us on a voyage where the aromatic essence of Lemon Dill Baked Cod transcends the limitations of health-conscious dining, proving that nourishment can be a celebration. This isn't just a cookbook; it's a testament to the idea that restriction doesn't mean resignation, and healthful meals can be a gourmet experience.

So, turn the page, tie your apron, and let the adventure begin. "The Renal Rejuvenation Cookbook" isn't just a collection of recipes; it's a passport to a culinary realm where kidney health and culinary delight coalesce, creating a symphony of flavors that echo the harmony of a well-nourished life.

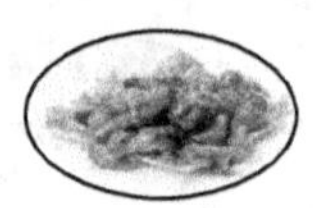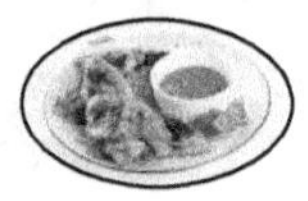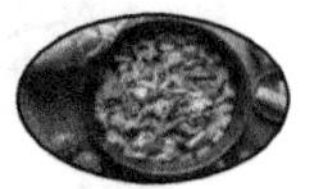

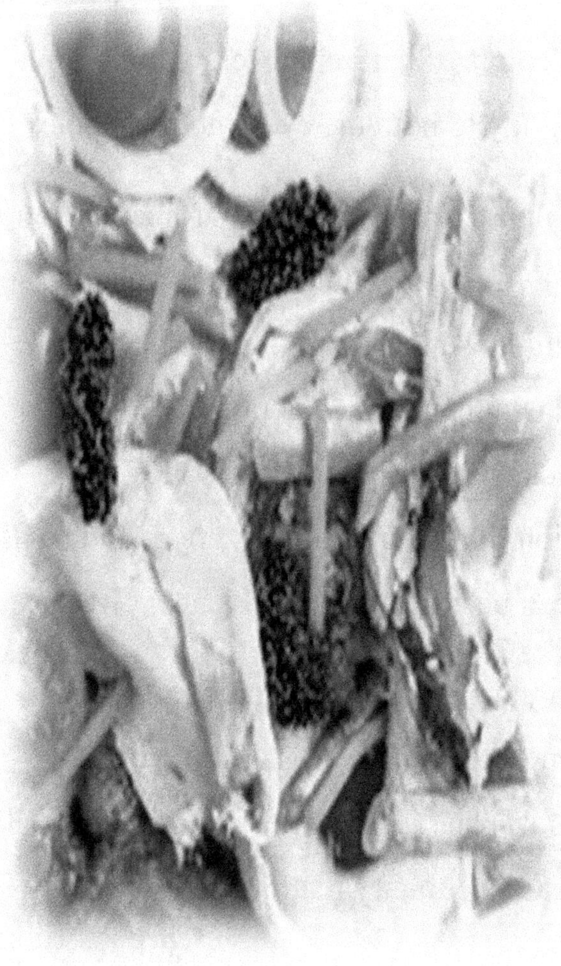

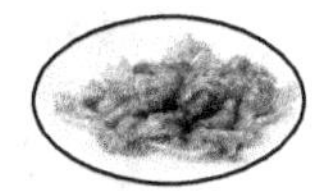 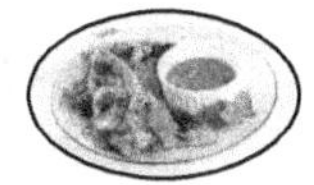 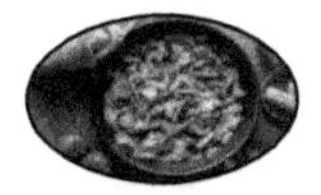

1. GRILLED LEMON HERB CHICKEN

Ingredients:

- 4 boneless, skinless chicken breasts

- 2 tablespoons olive oil

- 2 teaspoons dried oregano

- 1 teaspoon dried thyme

- 1 teaspoon garlic powder

- 1/2 teaspoon salt

- 1/4 teaspoon black pepper

- Juice of 1 lemon

- Fresh parsley (for garnish)

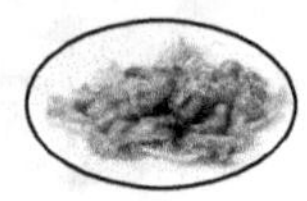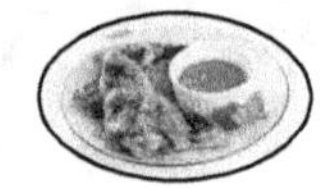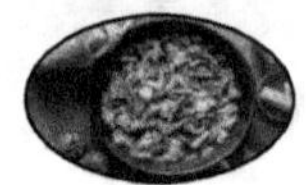

Instructions:

1. Preheat the grill to medium-high heat.

2. In a small bowl, mix together olive oil, oregano, thyme, garlic powder, salt, and black pepper to create a marinade.

3. Brush the chicken breasts with the marinade and place them on the grill.

4. Grill for 6-8 minutes per side or until the internal temperature reaches 165°F (74°C).

5. Squeeze lemon juice over the grilled chicken before serving.

6. Garnish with fresh parsley.

2. Herb-Roasted Salmon

Ingredients:

- 4 salmon fillets–

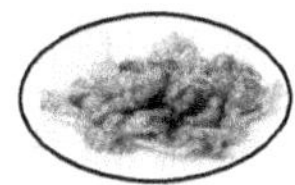 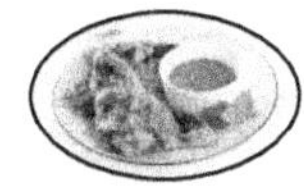 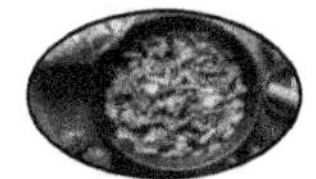

- 2 tablespoons olive oil

- 1 teaspoon dried rosemary

- 1 teaspoon dried thyme

- 1/2 teaspoon garlic powder

- 1/2 teaspoon onion powder

- 1/4 teaspoon salt

- 1/4 teaspoon black pepper

- Lemon wedges (for serving)

Instructions:

1. Preheat the oven to 400°F (200°C).

2. Arrange the salmon fillets on a parchment paper-lined baking sheet.

3. In a small bowl, mix olive oil, rosemary, thyme, garlic powder, onion powder, salt, and black pepper.

4. Brush the salmon fillets with the herb mixture.

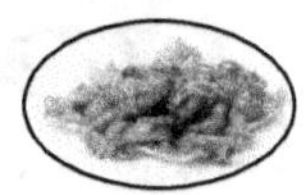 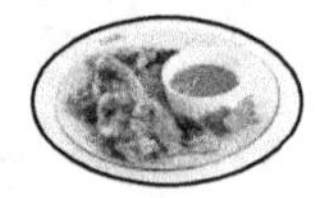 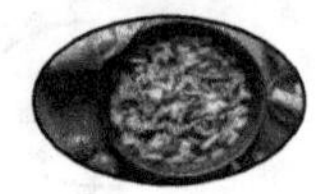

5. Roast in the oven for 12-15 minutes or until the salmon flakes easily with a fork.

6. Serve with lemon wedges on the side.

3. QUINOA AND VEGETABLE STIR-FRY

Ingredients:

- 1 cup quinoa, rinsed

- Two cups of mixed veggies, such as carrots, bell peppers, and broccoli

- 2 tablespoons low-sodium soy sauce

- 1 tablespoon olive oil

- 1 teaspoon grated ginger

- 2 cloves garlic, minced

- 1/4 cup chopped green onions

- Sesame seeds (for garnish)—

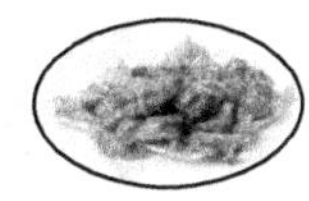 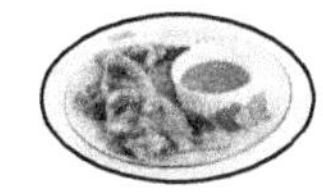 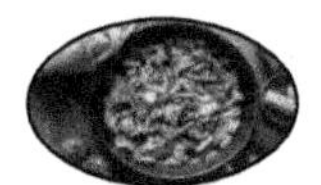

Instructions:

1. Cook quinoa according to package instructions.

2. In a large skillet, heat olive oil over medium heat.

3. Add ginger and garlic, sauté for 1 minute.

4. Add mixed vegetables and cook until tender-crisp.

5. Stir in cooked quinoa and soy sauce, tossing to combine.

6. Add sesame seeds and chopped green onions as garnish.

4. TURKEY AND VEGETABLE CHILI

Ingredients:

- 1 lb ground turkey

- 1 onion, diced

- 2 bell peppers, chopped

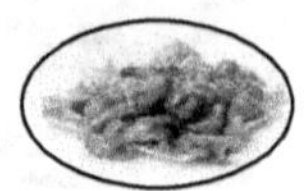 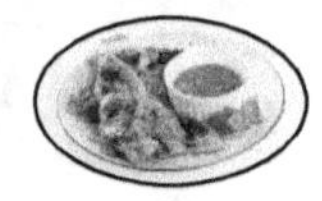 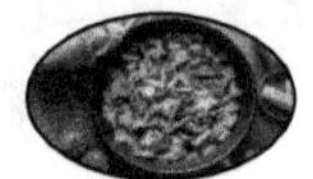

- 2 cloves garlic, minced

- One can (15 oz) of drained low-sodium kidney beans

- 1 can (15 oz) diced tomatoes

- 1 cup low-sodium chicken broth

- 2 teaspoons chili powder

- 1 teaspoon cumin

- 1/2 teaspoon paprika

- Salt and pepper to taste

Instructions:

1. In a large pot, brown ground turkey over medium heat.

2. Add onions, bell peppers, and garlic; sauté until vegetables are softened.

3. Stir in kidney beans, diced tomatoes, chicken broth, chili powder, cumin, paprika, salt, and pepper.

4. Simmer for 20-25 minutes, stirring occasionally.–

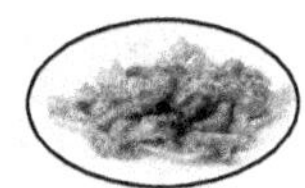 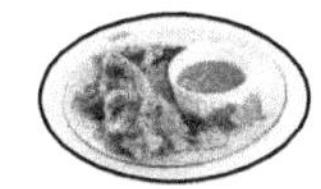 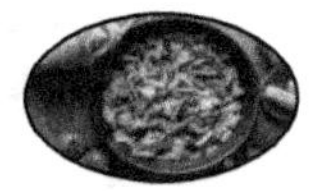

5. Baked Lemon Garlic Tilapia

Ingredients:

- 4 tilapia fillets

- 2 tablespoons olive oil

- 2 cloves garlic, minced

- 1 teaspoon dried thyme

- 1/2 teaspoon paprika

- 1/4 teaspoon salt

- 1/4 teaspoon black pepper

- Zest and juice of 1 lemon

Instructions:

1. Preheat the oven to 375°F (190°C).

2. Place tilapia fillets on a baking sheet lined with parchment paper.

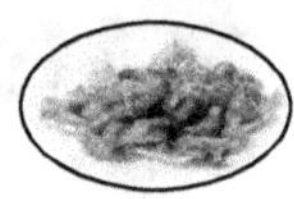 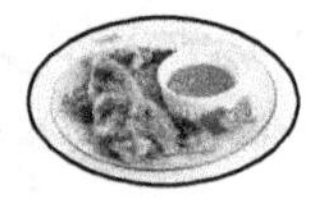 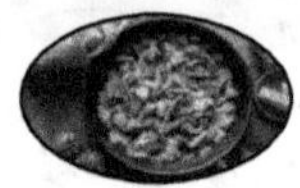

3. In a small bowl, mix olive oil, garlic, thyme, paprika, salt, pepper, lemon zest, and lemon juice.

4. Brush the tilapia fillets with the lemon-garlic mixture.

5. Bake for 15-18 minutes or until the tilapia is opaque and flakes easily.

6. Vegetable and Lentil Soup

Ingredients:

- One cup of rinsed dried green or brown lentils

- 1 onion, diced

- 2 carrots, chopped

- 2 celery stalks, chopped

- 2 cloves garlic, minced–

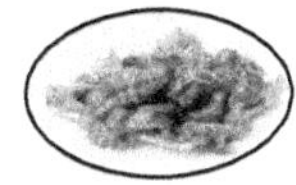 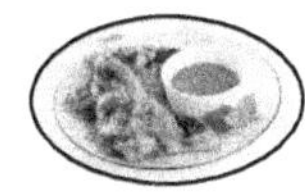 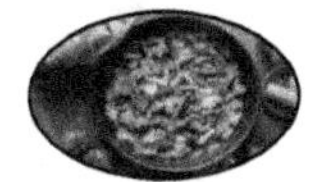

- 1 can (15 oz) diced tomatoes

- 6 cups low-sodium vegetable broth

- 1 teaspoon dried thyme

- 1/2 teaspoon cumin

- Salt and pepper to taste

- Fresh parsley (for garnish)

Instructions:

1. In a large pot, combine lentils, onion, carrots, celery, garlic, diced tomatoes, vegetable broth, thyme, cumin, salt, and pepper.

2. Bring to a boil, then reduce heat and simmer for 25-30 minutes or until lentils are tender.

3. Garnish with fresh parsley before serving.

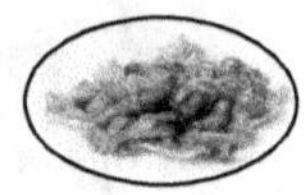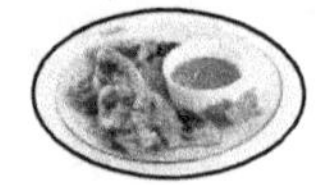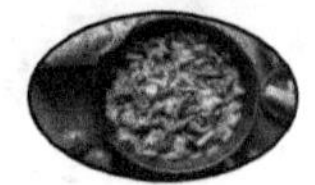

7. Spinach and Feta Stuffed Chicken Breast

Ingredients:

- 4 boneless, skinless chicken breasts

- 2 cups fresh spinach, chopped

- 1/2 cup feta cheese, crumbled

- 2 tablespoons olive oil

- 1 teaspoon dried oregano

- 1/2 teaspoon garlic powder

- Salt and pepper to taste

Instructions:

1. Preheat the oven to 400°F (200°C).

2. In a mixing bowl, combine chopped spinach, feta cheese, olive oil, oregano, garlic powder, salt, and pepper.

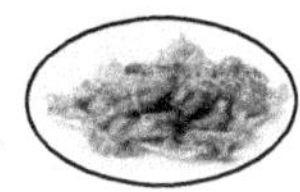 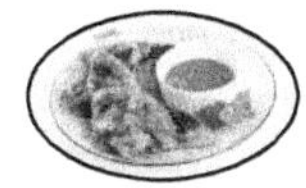 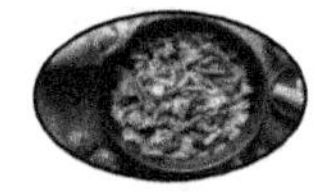

3. .Cut a pocket in each chicken breast by making a horizontal slit in it.

4. Stuff each pocket with the spinach and feta mixture.

5. Bake for 25-30 minutes or until the chicken is cooked through.

8. Mango Salsa Shrimp Tacos

Ingredients:

- 1 lb shrimp, peeled and deveined

- 2 mangos, diced

- 1/2 red onion, finely chopped

- 1 jalapeño, seeded and diced

- 1/4 cup fresh cilantro, chopped

- 2 tablespoons lime juice

- 8 small corn tortillas

- Cabbage slaw (optional)

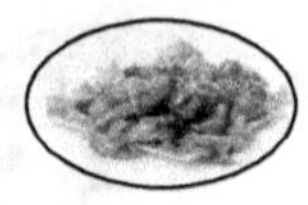 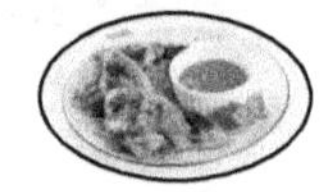 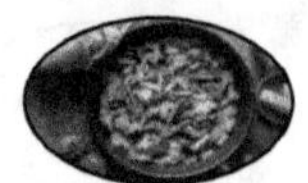

Instructions:

1. In a bowl, combine shrimp, diced mango, red onion, jalapeño, cilantro, and lime juice.

2. Marinate for 15 minutes.

3. Heat a skillet over medium-high heat and cook shrimp for 2-3 minutes per side.

4. Warm corn tortillas and fill with shrimp mixture.

5. Top with cabbage slaw if desired.

9. Eggplant and Tomato Casserole

Ingredients:

- 1 large eggplant, sliced

- 2 cups cherry tomatoes, halved

- 1 onion, sliced

- 2 cloves garlic, minced

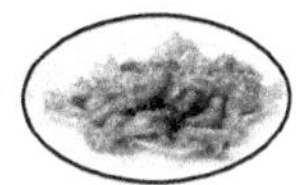 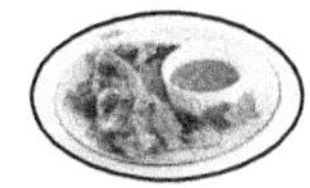 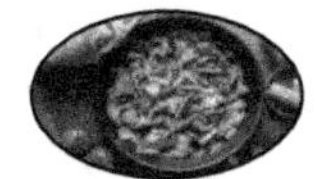

- 2 tablespoons olive oil

- 1 teaspoon dried basil

- 1/2 teaspoon dried oregano

- Salt and pepper to taste

- 1/2 cup grated Parmesan cheese

Instructions:

1. Preheat the oven to 375°F (190°C).

2. In a baking dish, layer sliced eggplant, cherry tomatoes, and sliced onions.

3. In a bowl, mix minced garlic, olive oil, basil, oregano, salt, and pepper.

4. Drizzle the olive oil mixture over the vegetables and toss to coat.

5. Sprinkle Parmesan cheese on top.

6. Bake for 30-35 minutes or until the vegetables are tender.–

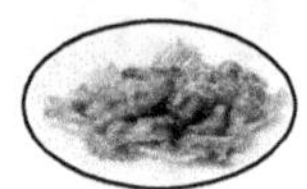 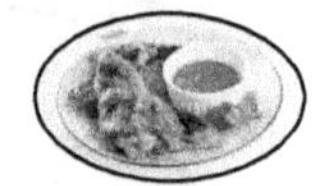 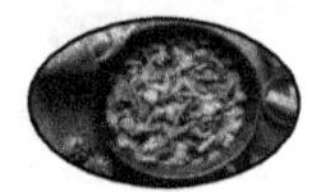

10. Lemon Dill Baked Cod

Ingredients:

- 4 cod fillets

- 2 tablespoons olive oil

- 1 tablespoon fresh dill, chopped

- 2 cloves garlic, minced

- 1 lemon, sliced

- Salt and pepper to taste

Instructions:

1. Preheat the oven to 400°F (200°C).

2. Place cod fillets on a baking sheet lined with parchment paper.

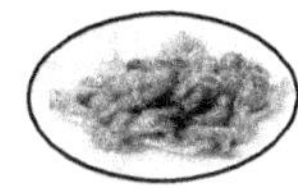 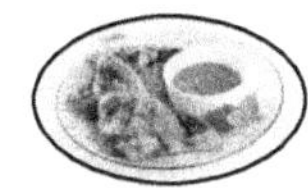 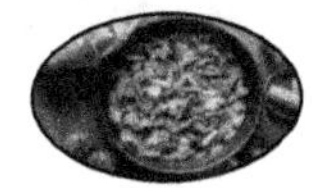

3. In a small bowl, mix olive oil, dill, garlic, salt, and pepper.

4. Brush the cod fillets with the olive oil mixture.

5. Top each fillet with a slice of lemon.

6. Bake for 15-18 minutes or until the cod is opaque and flakes easily.

11. VEGETARIAN CHICKPEA SALAD

Ingredients:

- Two cans of rinsed and drained chickpeas, 15 ounces each

- 1 cucumber, diced

- 1 bell pepper, diced

- 1/2 red onion, finely chopped

- 1 cup cherry tomatoes, halved

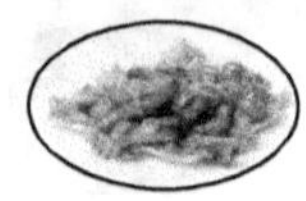 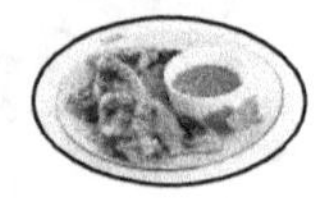 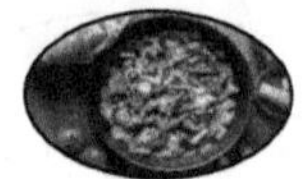

- 1/4 cup fresh parsley, chopped

- 3 tablespoons olive oil

- 2 tablespoons red wine vinegar

- 1 teaspoon dried oregano

- Salt and pepper to taste

Instructions:

1. In a large bowl, combine chickpeas, cucumber, bell pepper, red onion, cherry tomatoes, and parsley.

2. Combine the olive oil, red wine vinegar, oregano, salt, and pepper in a small bowl.

3. Pour the dressing over the salad and toss until well combined.–

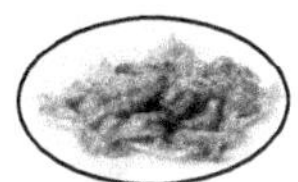 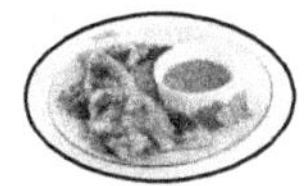 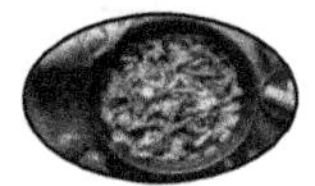

12. Cauliflower Rice Pilaf

Ingredients:

- 1 head cauliflower, riced

- 2 tablespoons olive oil

- 1 onion, finely chopped

- 2 cloves garlic, minced

- 1/2 cup low-sodium vegetable broth

- 1/4 cup sliced almonds

- 1/4 cup fresh cilantro, chopped

- Salt and pepper to taste

Instructions:

1. In a food processor, pulse cauliflower until it resembles rice.–

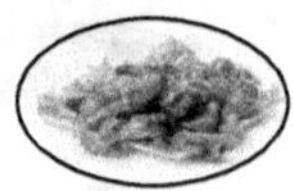 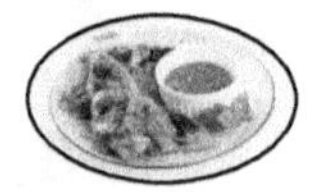 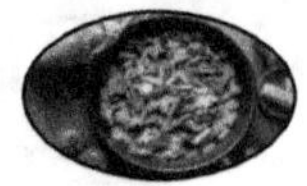

2. In a large skillet, heat olive oil over medium heat.

3. Sauté onion and garlic until softened.

4. Add cauliflower rice and cook for 5-7 minutes.

5. Pour in vegetable broth and continue cooking until the cauliflower is tender.

6. Stir in sliced almonds and cilantro. Season with salt and pepper.

13. Sweet Potato and Black Bean Tacos

Ingredients:

- 2 sweet potatoes, peeled and diced

- One can (15 ounces) of rinsed and drained black beans

- 1 teaspoon ground cumin

- 1/2 teaspoon chili powder

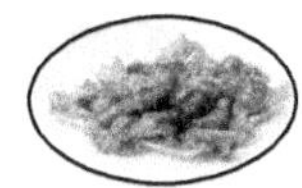 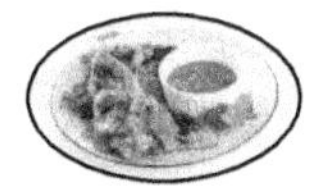 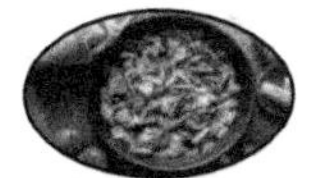

- 1/4 teaspoon cayenne pepper

- 8 small whole wheat tortillas

- Avocado slices (for serving)

- Fresh cilantro (for garnish)

Instructions:

1. Steam or boil sweet potatoes until fork-tender.

2. In a bowl, combine sweet potatoes, black beans, cumin, chili powder, and cayenne pepper.

3. Warm tortillas and fill with the sweet potato and black bean mixture.

4. Top with avocado slices and garnish with fresh cilantro.–

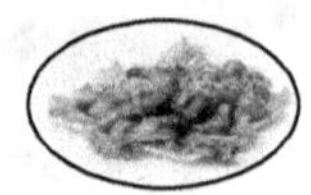 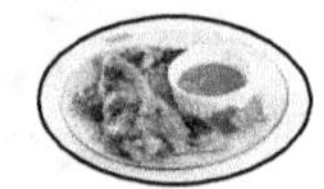 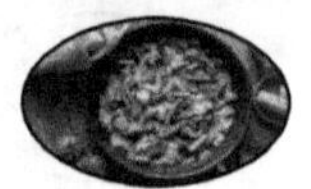

14. Turkey and Vegetable Skewers

Ingredients:

- A one-pound turkey breast, cubed

- 1 zucchini, sliced

- 1 red onion, cut into chunks

- Cherry tomatoes

- 2 tablespoons olive oil

- 1 teaspoon dried thyme

- 1 teaspoon paprika

- Salt and pepper to taste

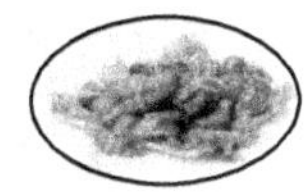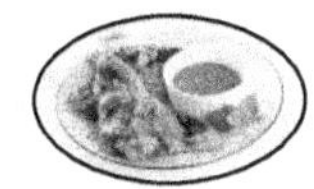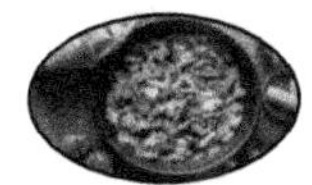

Instructions:

1. Preheat the grill to medium-high heat.

2. Thread turkey cubes, zucchini slices, red onion chunks, and cherry tomatoes onto skewers.

3. In a small bowl, mix olive oil, thyme, paprika, salt, and pepper.

4. Apply the olive oil mixture to the skewers.

5. Grill for 10-12 minutes, turning occasionally, until the turkey is cooked through.

15. CREAMY ASPARAGUS RISOTTO

Ingredients:

- 1 cup Arborio rice

- 1 bunch asparagus, trimmed and chopped–

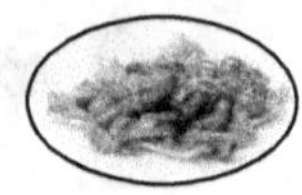 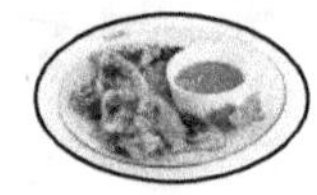 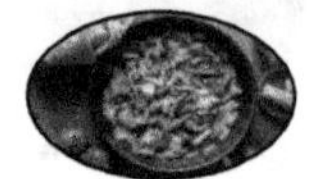

- 1 onion, finely chopped

- 2 cloves garlic, minced

- 4 cups low-sodium vegetable broth, warmed

- 1/2 cup dry white wine

- 1/4 cup grated Parmesan cheese

- 2 tablespoons olive oil

- Salt and pepper to taste

Instructions:

1. In a large skillet, sauté onion and garlic in olive oil until translucent.

2. Add Arborio rice and cook for 2 minutes.

3. Pour in white wine and cook until mostly evaporated.

4. Gradually add warm vegetable broth, stirring constantly, until the rice is creamy and cooked al dente.

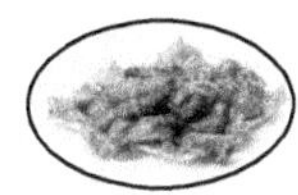 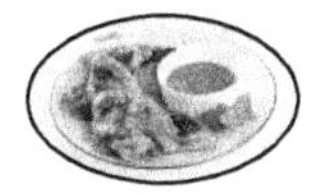 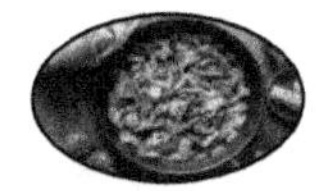

5. Stir in asparagus and Parmesan cheese. Season with
    salt and pepper.

16. Chicken and Vegetable Curry

Ingredients:

- 1 lb boneless, skinless chicken thighs, cut into cubes

- 1 eggplant, diced

- 1 bell pepper, sliced

- 1 onion, chopped

- 2 cloves garlic, minced

- 1 can (14 oz) coconut milk

- 2 tablespoons curry powder

- 1 teaspoon ground turmeric

- 1 teaspoon ground cumin

- 1/2 teaspoon cayenne pepper

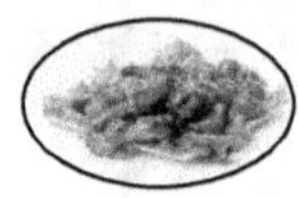 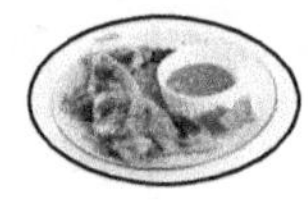 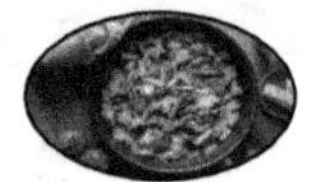

- Fresh cilantro (for garnish)

- Brown rice (for serving)

Instructions:

1. In a large pot, brown chicken cubes over medium heat.

2. Add eggplant, bell pepper, onion, and garlic; sauté until vegetables are softened.

3. Stir in coconut milk, curry powder, turmeric, cumin, and cayenne pepper.

4. Simmer for 20-25 minutes, stirring occasionally.

5. Garnish with fresh cilantro and serve over brown rice.–

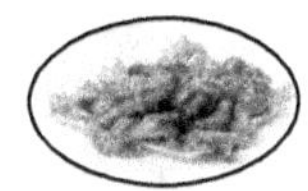 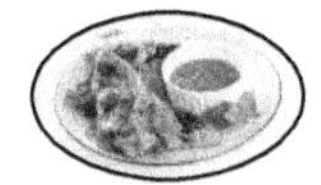 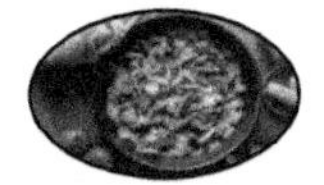

17. Shrimp and Broccoli Stir-Fry

Ingredients:

- 1 lb shrimp, peeled and deveined

- 4 cups broccoli florets

- 1 red bell pepper, sliced

- 2 tablespoons low-sodium soy sauce

- 1 tablespoon honey

- 1 tablespoon sesame oil

- 2 cloves garlic, minced

- 1 teaspoon grated ginger

- Brown rice (for serving)–

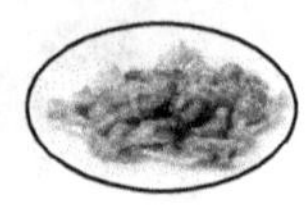 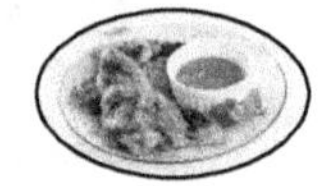 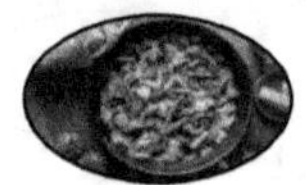

Instructions:

1. In a wok or large skillet, stir-fry shrimp until pink and opaque. Remove from pan.

2. Stir-fry broccoli and bell pepper until crisp-tender.

3. In a small bowl, whisk together soy sauce, honey, sesame oil, garlic, and ginger.

4. Return shrimp to the pan and pour the sauce over the mixture. Cook until heated through.

5. Serve over brown rice.

18. MUSHROOM AND SPINACH STUFFED BELL PEPPERS

Ingredients:–

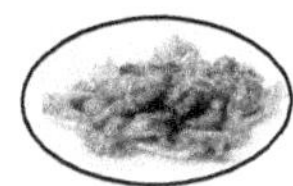 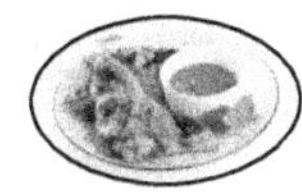 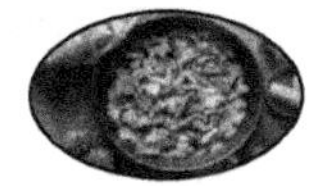

- Four bell peppers, cut in half and seeded

- 2 cups mushrooms, finely chopped

- 2 cups fresh spinach, chopped

- 1 onion, diced

- 2 cloves garlic, minced

- 1 cup cooked quinoa

- 1/2 cup low-sodium vegetable broth

- 1 teaspoon dried thyme

- 1/2 teaspoon smoked paprika

- Salt and pepper to taste

- Grated mozzarella cheese (optional)

Instructions:

1. Preheat the oven to 375°F (190°C).

2. In a skillet, sauté mushrooms, spinach, onion, and garlic until vegetables are softened.

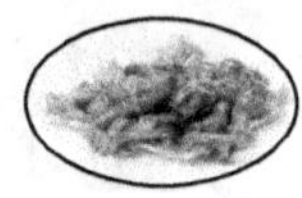 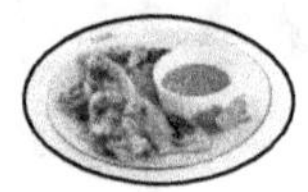 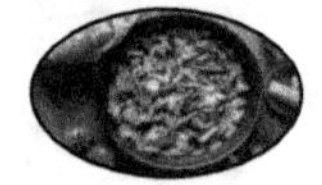

3. Stir in cooked quinoa, vegetable broth, thyme, paprika, salt, and pepper.

4. Fill each bell pepper half with the quinoa mixture.

5. Optionally, sprinkle grated mozzarella cheese on top.

6. Bake for 25-30 minutes or until the peppers are tender.

19. Lentil and Vegetable Curry Soup

Ingredients:

- One cup of rinsed dried green or brown lentils

- 2 carrots, diced

- 2 celery stalks, chopped

- 1 onion, chopped–

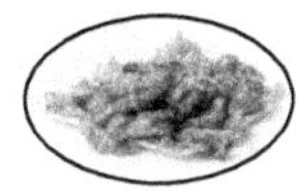 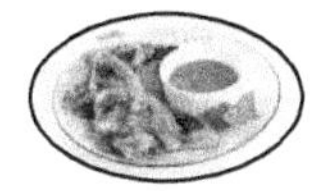 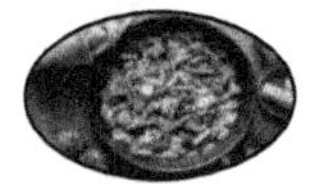

- 2 cloves garlic, minced

- 1 can (14 oz) diced tomatoes

- 6 cups low-sodium vegetable broth

- 2 tablespoons curry powder

- 1 teaspoon ground cumin

- Salt and pepper to taste

- Fresh cilantro (for garnish)

Instructions:

1. In a large pot, combine lentils, carrots, celery, onion, garlic, diced tomatoes, vegetable broth, curry powder, cumin, salt, and pepper.

2. Bring to a boil, then reduce heat and simmer for 25-30 minutes or until lentils are tender.

3. Garnish with fresh cilantro before serving.–

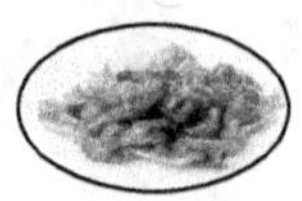 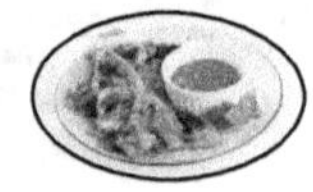 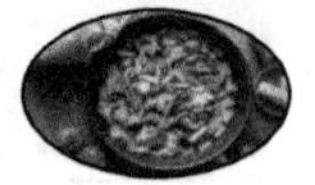

20. Tofu and Vegetable Stir-Fry

Ingredients:

- 1 block firm tofu, cubed

- 2 cups broccoli florets

- 1 bell pepper, sliced

- 1 carrot, julienned

- 2 tablespoons low-sodium soy sauce

- 1 tablespoon hoisin sauce

- 1 tablespoon sesame oil

- 2 cloves garlic, minced

- 1 teaspoon grated ginger

- Green onions (for garnish)

- Brown rice (for serving)–

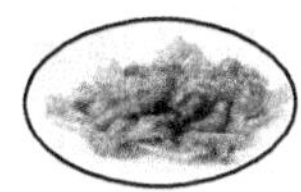 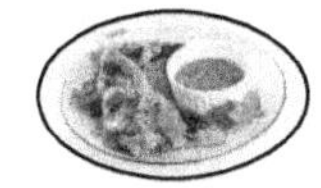 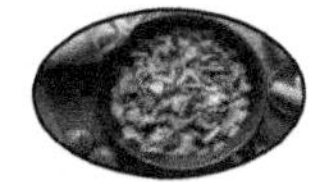

Instructions:

1. Press tofu to remove excess water, then cut into cubes.

2. In a wok or large skillet, stir-fry tofu until golden brown. Remove from pan.

3. Stir-fry broccoli, bell pepper, and carrot until crisp-tender.

4. In a small bowl, mix soy sauce, hoisin sauce, sesame oil, garlic, and ginger.

5. Return tofu to the pan and pour the sauce over the mixture. Cook until heated through.

6. Garnish with green onions and serve over brown rice.–

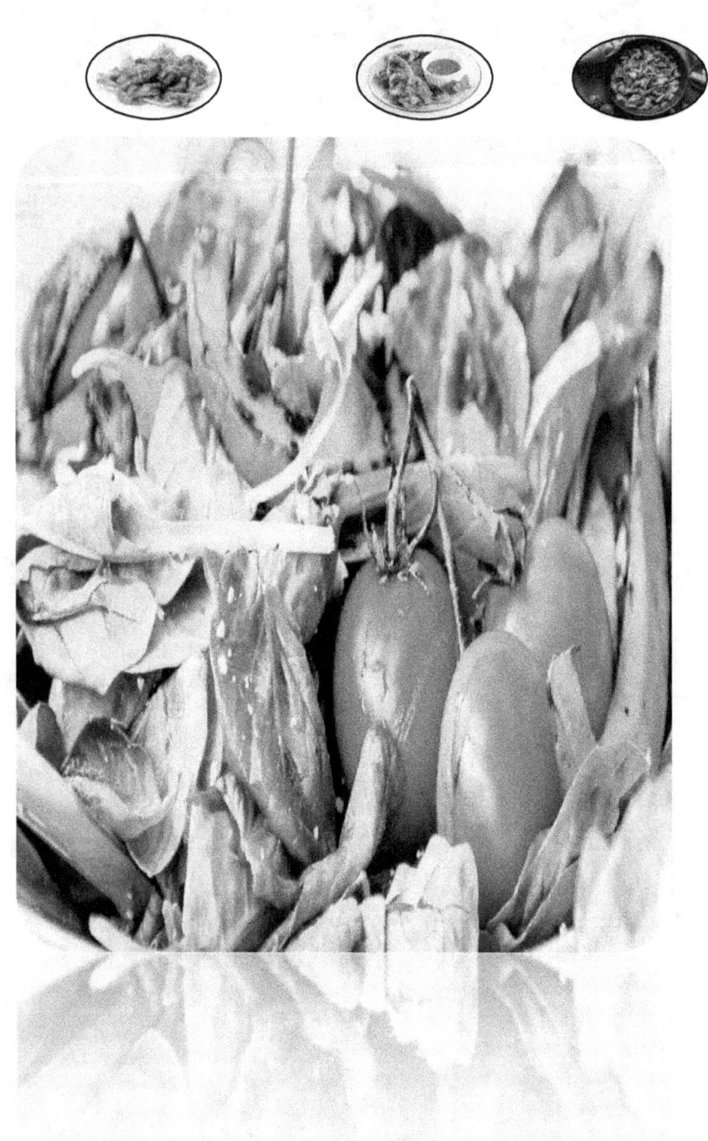

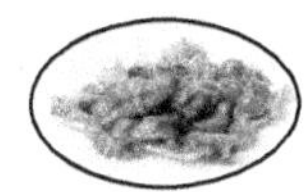 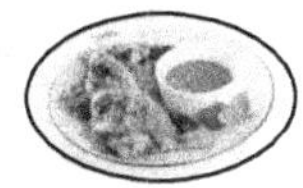 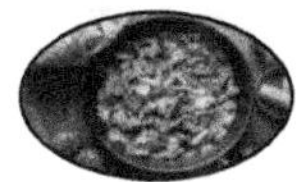

CONCLUSION

As we close the chapters of "The Renal Rejuvenation Cookbook," we reflect on the aromatic tales and flavorsome adventures that have unfolded. This culinary odyssey has been more than a collection of recipes; it's been a guide, a friend, and a beacon of healthful living.

In the tapestry of each dish, we've woven the threads of nourishment, flavor, and well-being. From the sizzling grills that birthed the Grilled Lemon Herb Chicken to the aromatic embrace of the Creamy Asparagus Risotto, our journey through these pages has been a celebration of the infinite possibilities within a renal-friendly kitchen.

Yet, as we bid adieu, let us not forget that this is not the end but a commencement. A commencement of a lifestyle where the kitchen is not a battlefield but a sanctuary, and every meal is an opportunity to nurture our bodies and souls. The recipes within this book are not mere instructions; they are

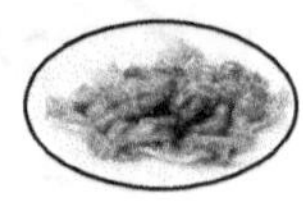 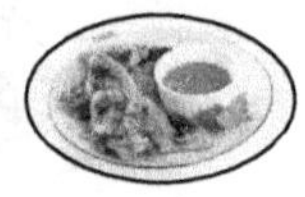 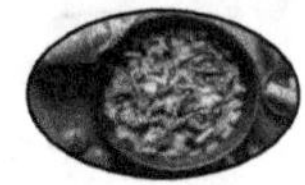

invitations to a dance, where the ingredients harmonize, and the outcome is a symphony of well-being.

May the echoes of these recipes resonate in your kitchens, reminding you that health need not be a compromise on flavor. As you embrace the art of renal rejuvenation, may your culinary endeavors be filled with joy, and may your plates be canvases of vibrant, healthful living.

Here's to a future where every bite is a step towards renal wellness, and every recipe is a testament to the power of mindful, delicious cooking. As you savor the last morsels of our gastronomic journey, remember that this cookbook is not just a guide; it's a companion on your path to a healthier, more flavorful life.

Bon appétit, and may your journey towards renal health be as delectable as the recipes within these pages.

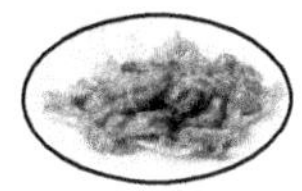 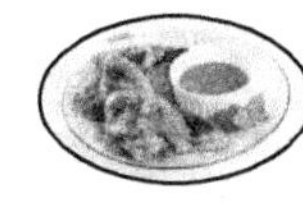 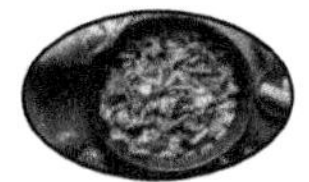

WE KNOW...

THAT'S WHY WE ARE SAYING THANK YOU...

"We know time is the unit of destiny, that's why we are saying thank you."

Dear Valued Customer,

we understand that time is a precious commodity, and we sincerely appreciate you choosing to spend a portion of it with us. Your decision to trust us with your purchase means the world to us, and we want to express our deepest gratitude.

Your support not only fuels our passion for delivering quality products but also contributes to the destiny of our business. Each customer is a vital part of our journey, and we are honored to have you

We strive to provide an exceptional shopping experience, and your satisfaction is our top priority. If you have any feedback or suggestions, we would love to hear from you. Your insights help us improve.

As a small token of our appreciation, we kindly invite you to share your experience by leaving a 5-star review. Your feedback not only boosts our morale but also assists fellow shoppers in making informed decisions.

Once again, thank you for choosing to buy this book. We look forward to serving you again and being a part of your destiny in the world of quality and excellence.

Warm regards,

Dr. Grace Hester–

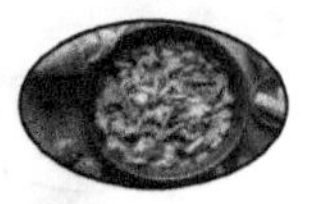
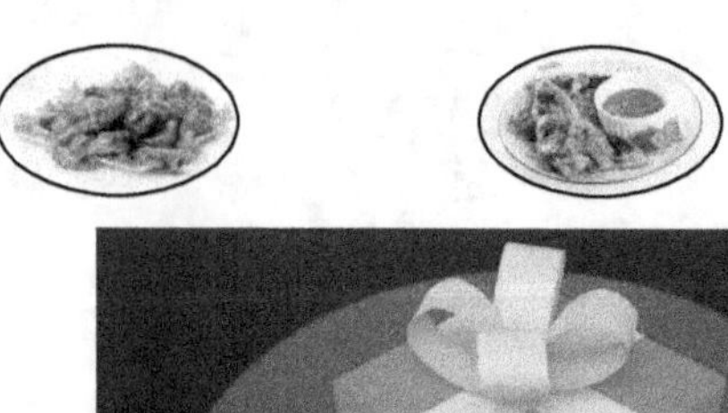

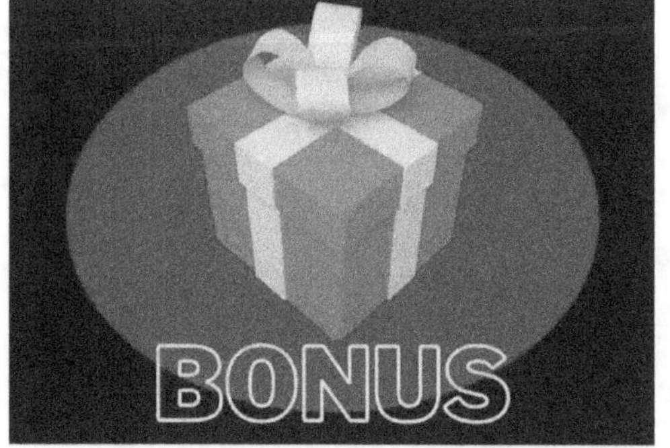

20 DAYS + MEAL PLANNER

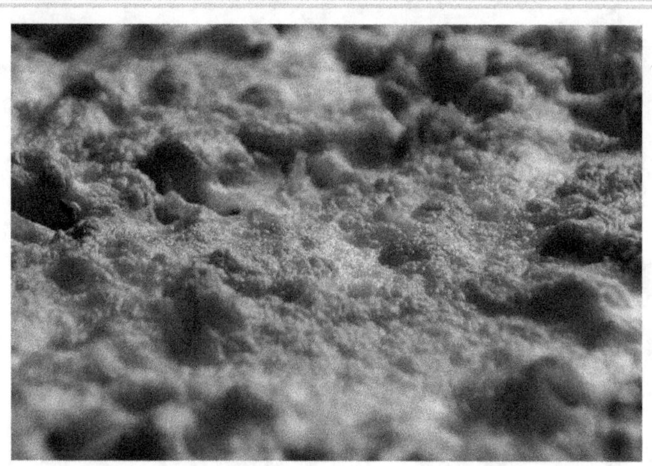

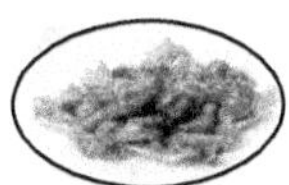 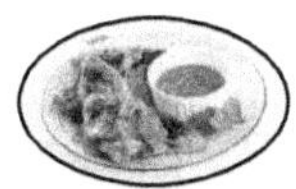 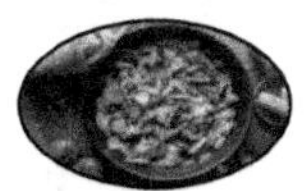

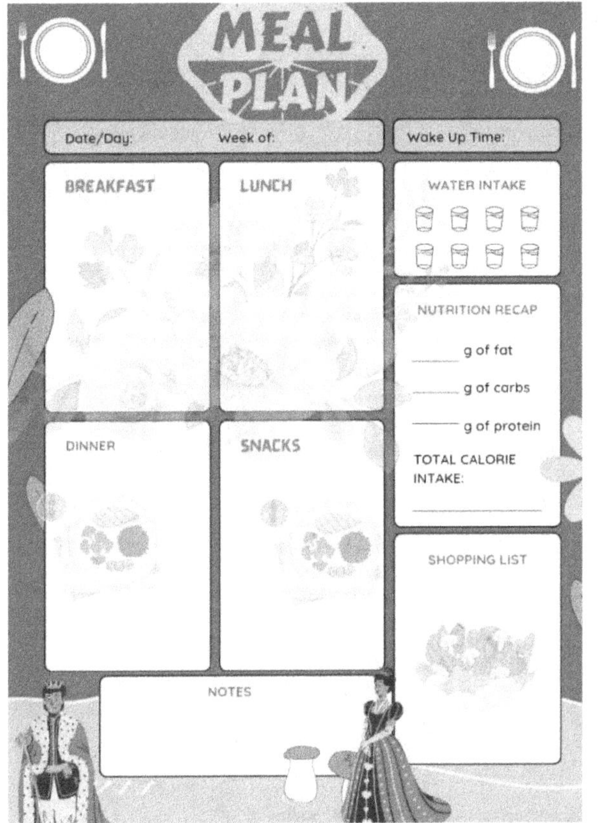

MEAL PLAN
Date/Day:
Week of:
Wake Up Time:
BREAKFAST
LUNCH
WATER INTAKE
NUTRITION RECAP
_______ g of fat
_______ g of carbs
_______ g of protein
TOTAL CALORIE INTAKE:
DINNER
SNACKS
SHOPPING LIST
NOTES

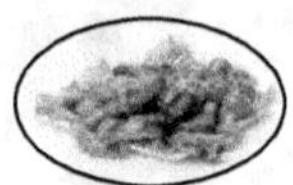 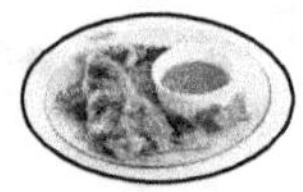 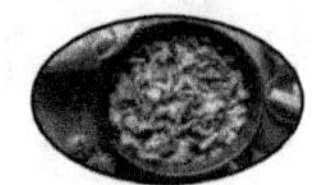

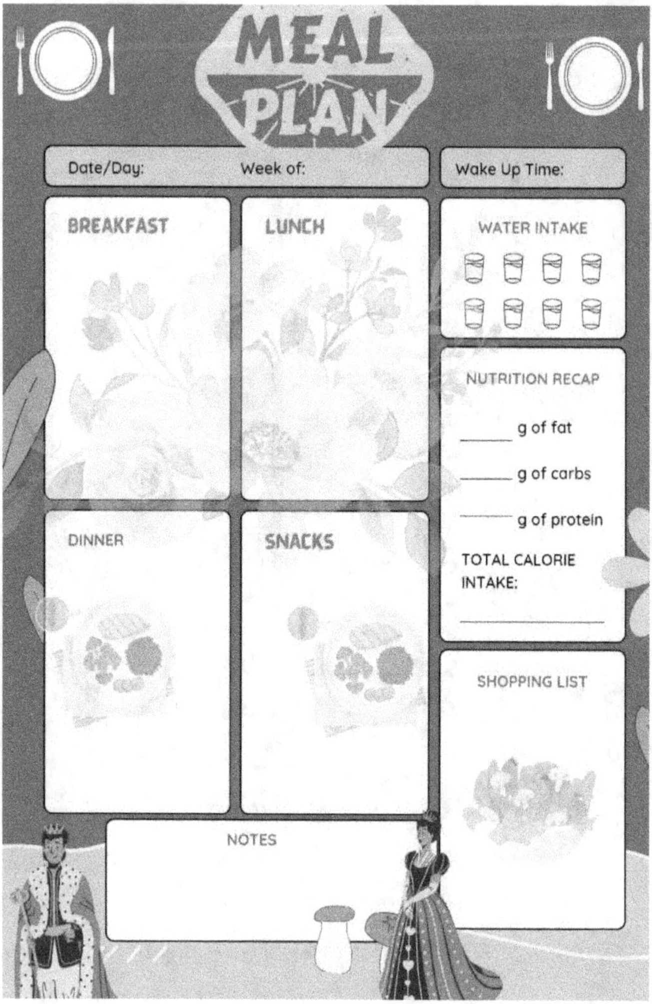

MEAL PLAN

| Date/Day: | Week of: | Wake Up Time: |

BREAKFAST

LUNCH

WATER INTAKE

NUTRITION RECAP

______ g of fat

______ g of carbs

______ g of protein

TOTAL CALORIE INTAKE:

____

DINNER

SNACKS

SHOPPING LIST

NOTES

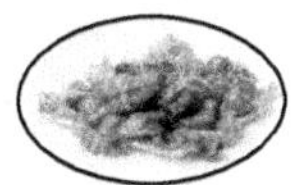 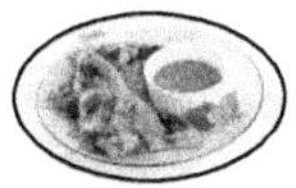 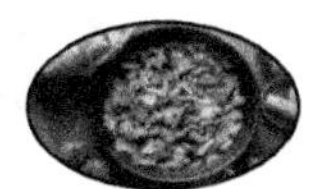

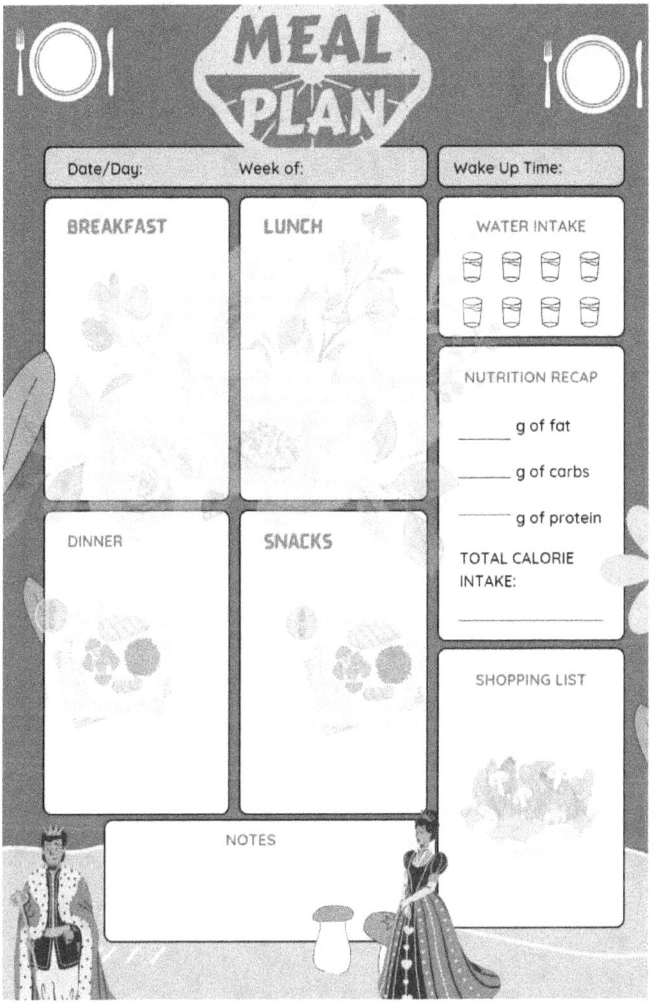

MEAL PLAN

Date/Day: | Week of: | Wake Up Time:

BREAKFAST

LUNCH

WATER INTAKE

NUTRITION RECAP

_______ g of fat

_______ g of carbs

_______ g of protein

TOTAL CALORIE INTAKE:

____

DINNER

SNACKS

SHOPPING LIST

NOTES

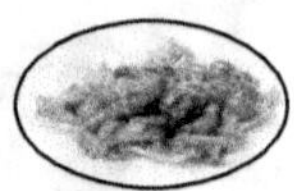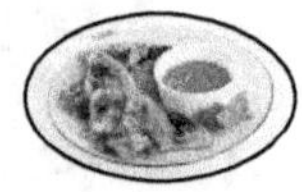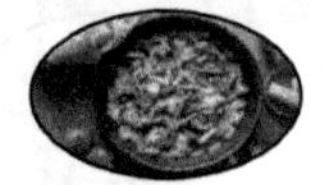

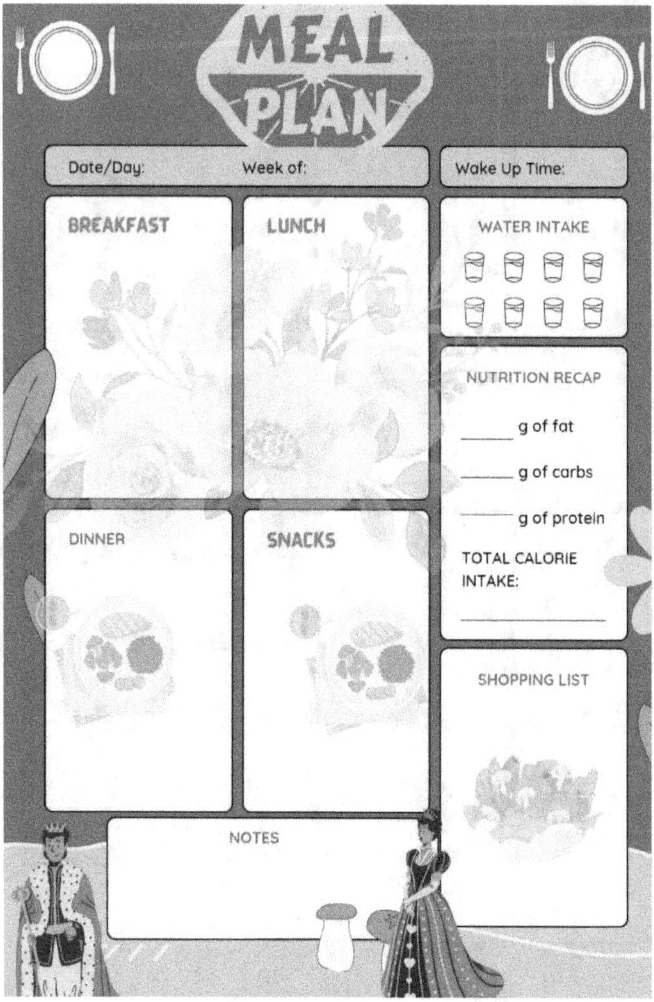

MEAL PLAN

| Date/Day: | Week of: | Wake Up Time: |

BREAKFAST

LUNCH

WATER INTAKE

NUTRITION RECAP

_______ g of fat

_______ g of carbs

_______ g of protein

TOTAL CALORIE INTAKE:

____

DINNER

SNACKS

SHOPPING LIST

NOTES

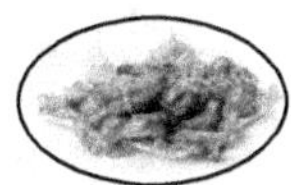 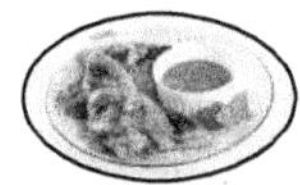 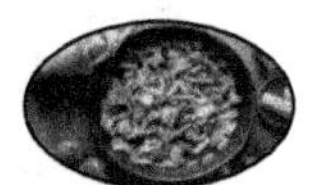

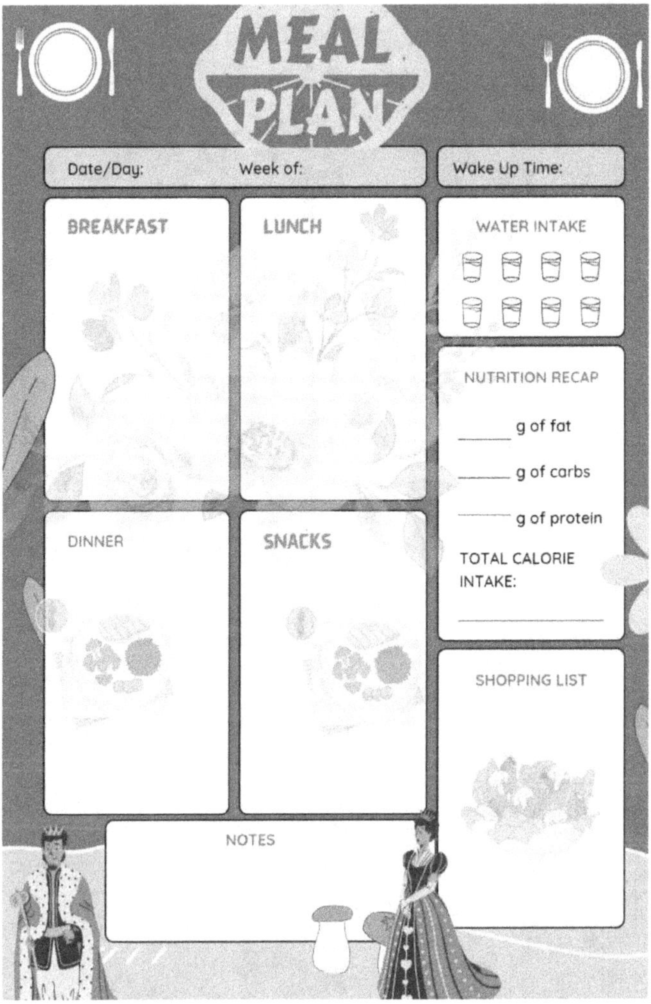

MEAL PLAN

Date/Day: Week of: Wake Up Time:

BREAKFAST

LUNCH

WATER INTAKE

NUTRITION RECAP

_______ g of fat

_______ g of carbs

_______ g of protein

TOTAL CALORIE INTAKE:

____

DINNER

SNACKS

SHOPPING LIST

NOTES

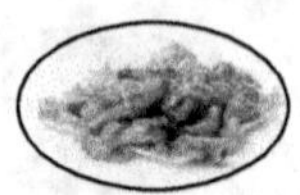 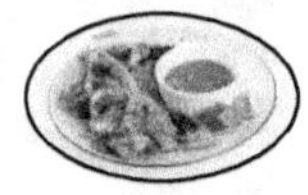 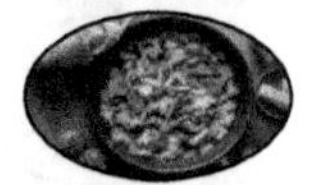

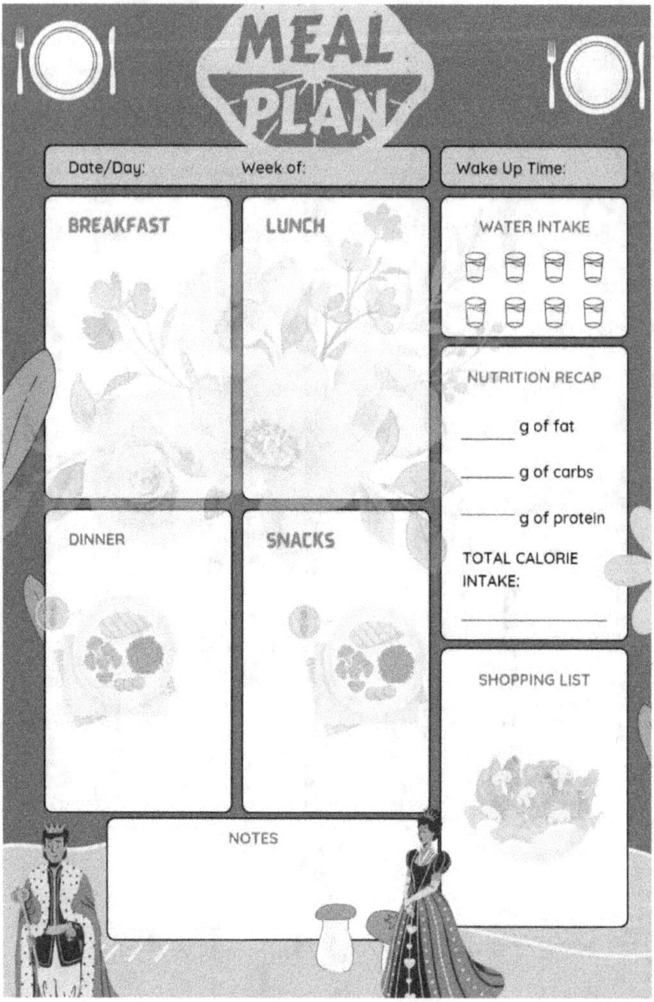

MEAL PLAN

Date/Day: | Week of: | Wake Up Time:

BREAKFAST

LUNCH

WATER INTAKE

NUTRITION RECAP

__________ g of fat

__________ g of carbs

__________ g of protein

TOTAL CALORIE INTAKE:

____

DINNER

SNACKS

SHOPPING LIST

NOTES

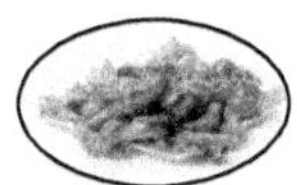 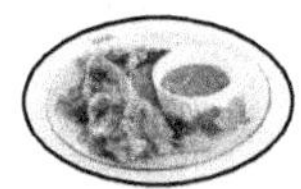 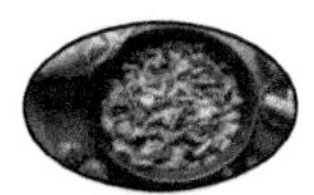

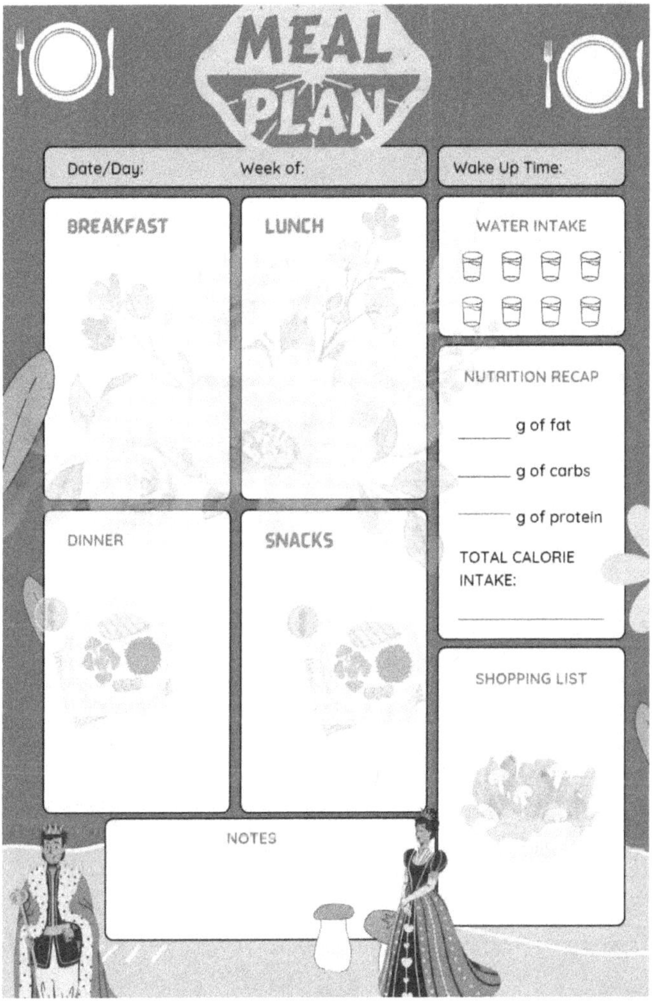

MEAL PLAN

| Date/Day: | Week of: | Wake Up Time: |

BREAKFAST

LUNCH

WATER INTAKE

NUTRITION RECAP

_______ g of fat

_______ g of carbs

_______ g of protein

TOTAL CALORIE INTAKE:

____

DINNER

SNACKS

SHOPPING LIST

NOTES

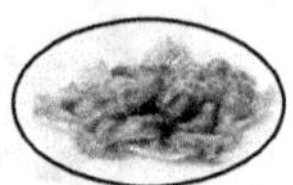
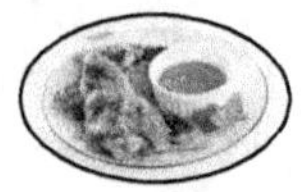
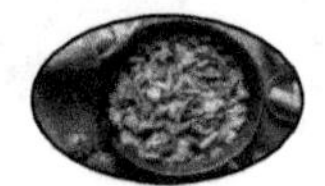

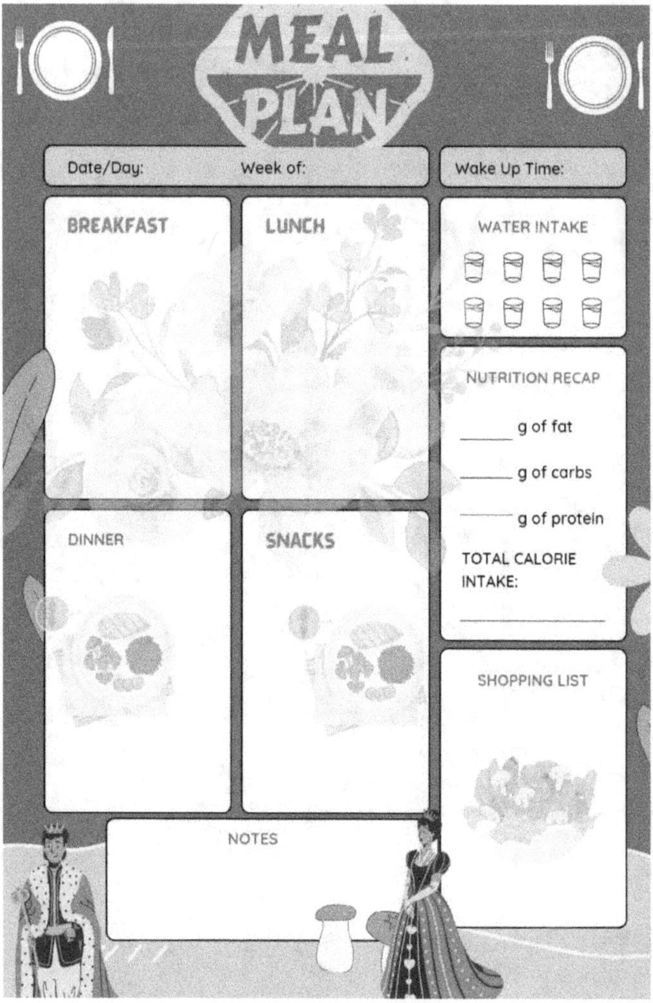

MEAL PLAN

| Date/Day: | Week of: | Wake Up Time: |

BREAKFAST

LUNCH

WATER INTAKE

NUTRITION RECAP

_______ g of fat

_______ g of carbs

_______ g of protein

TOTAL CALORIE INTAKE:

____

DINNER

SNACKS

SHOPPING LIST

NOTES

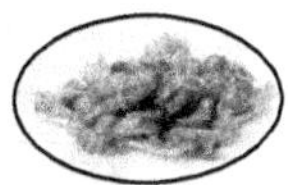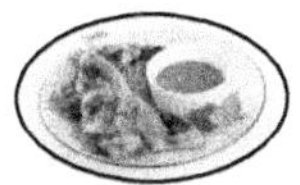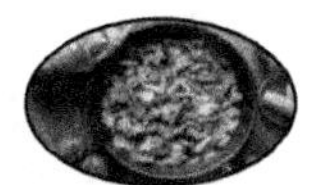

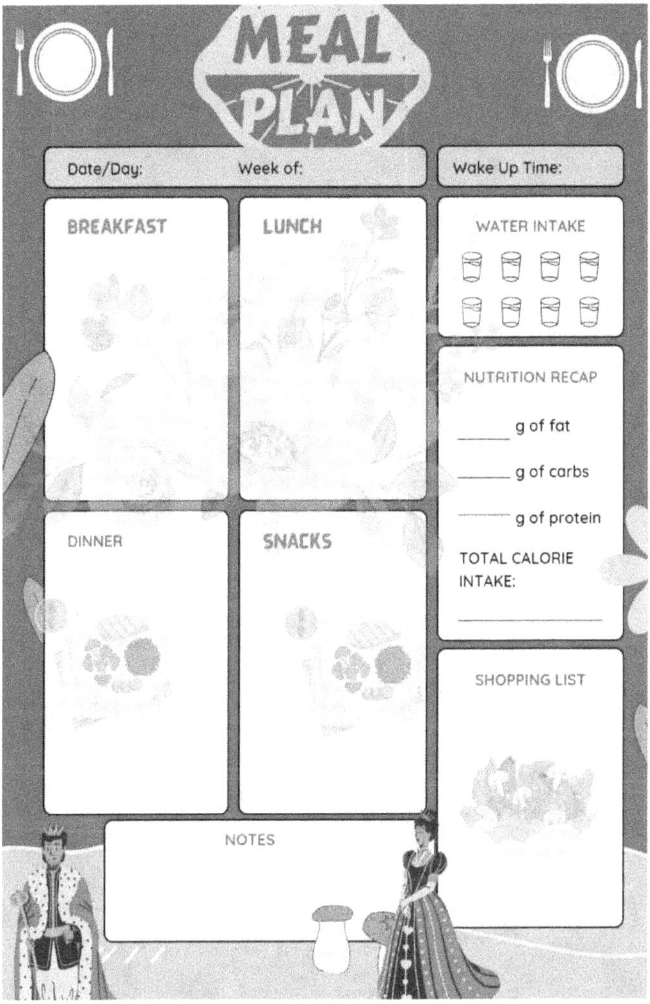

MEAL PLAN

| Date/Day: | Week of: | Wake Up Time: |

BREAKFAST

LUNCH

WATER INTAKE

NUTRITION RECAP

_______ g of fat

_______ g of carbs

_______ g of protein

TOTAL CALORIE INTAKE:

____

DINNER

SNACKS

SHOPPING LIST

NOTES

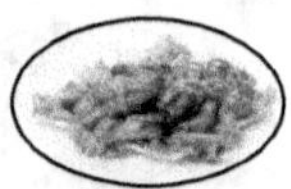 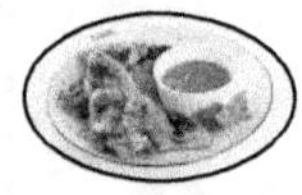 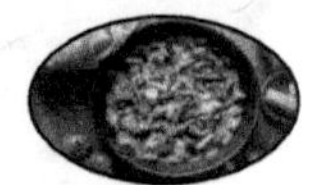

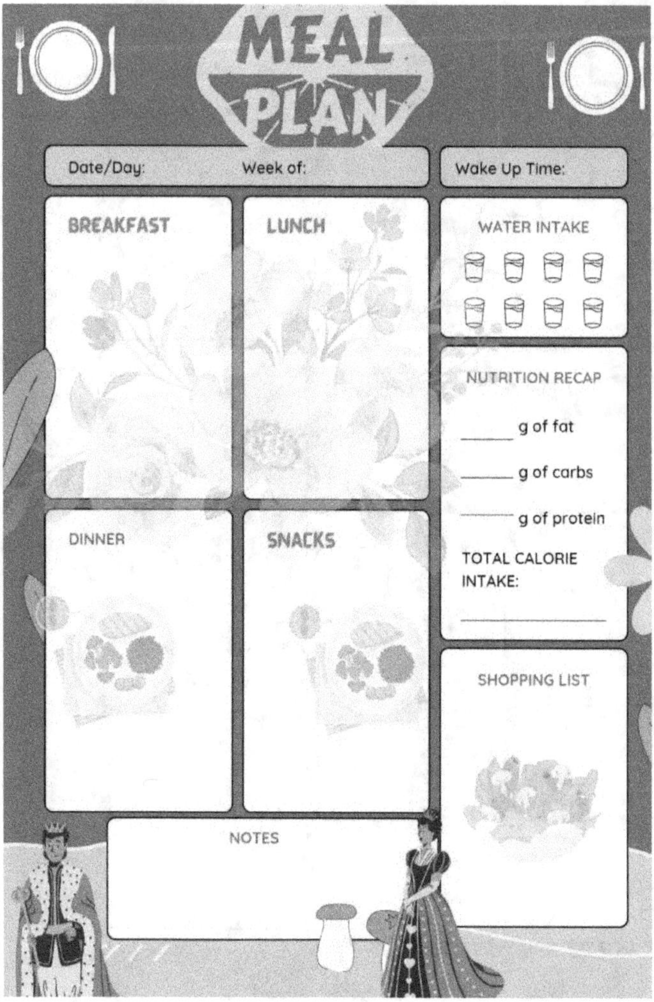

MEAL PLAN

Date/Day: Week of: Wake Up Time:

BREAKFAST

LUNCH

DINNER

SNACKS

WATER INTAKE

NUTRITION RECAP

________ g of fat

________ g of carbs

________ g of protein

TOTAL CALORIE INTAKE:

____

SHOPPING LIST

NOTES

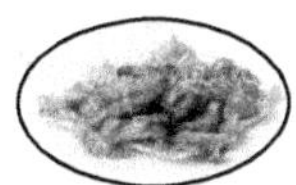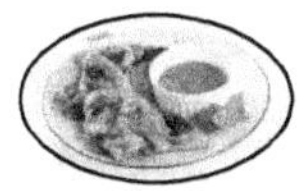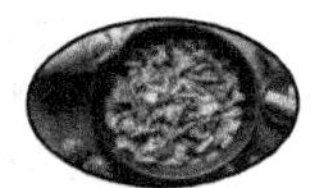

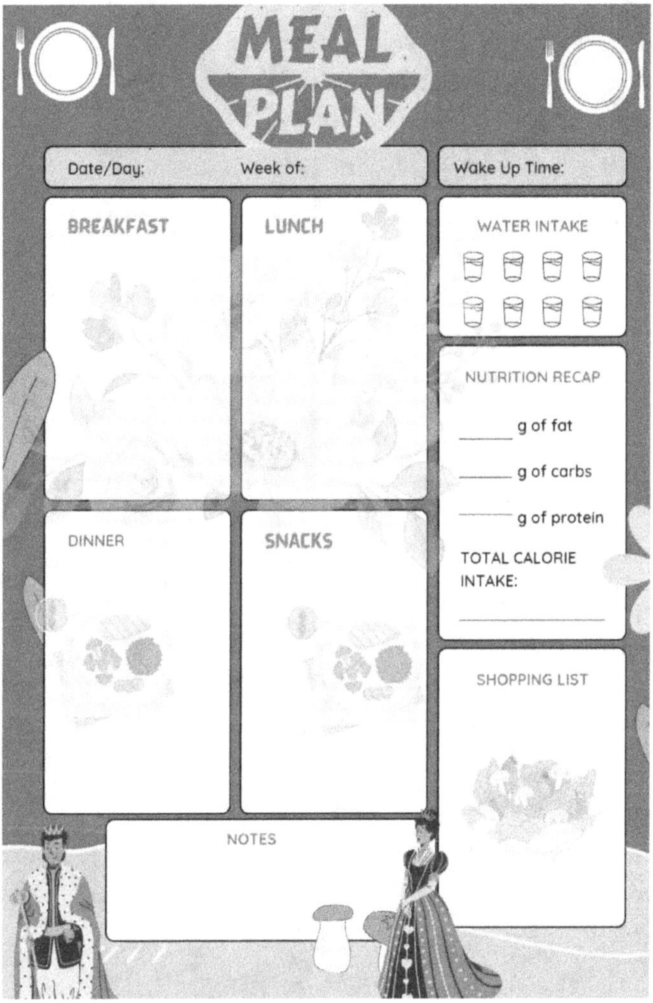

MEAL PLAN

Date/Day:	Week of:	Wake Up Time:

BREAKFAST

LUNCH

WATER INTAKE

NUTRITION RECAP

_________ g of fat

_________ g of carbs

_________ g of protein

TOTAL CALORIE INTAKE:

____

DINNER

SNACKS

SHOPPING LIST

NOTES

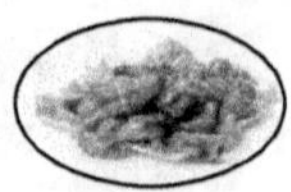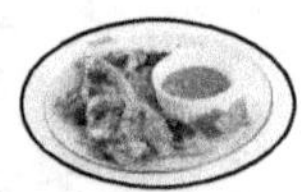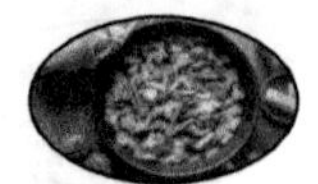

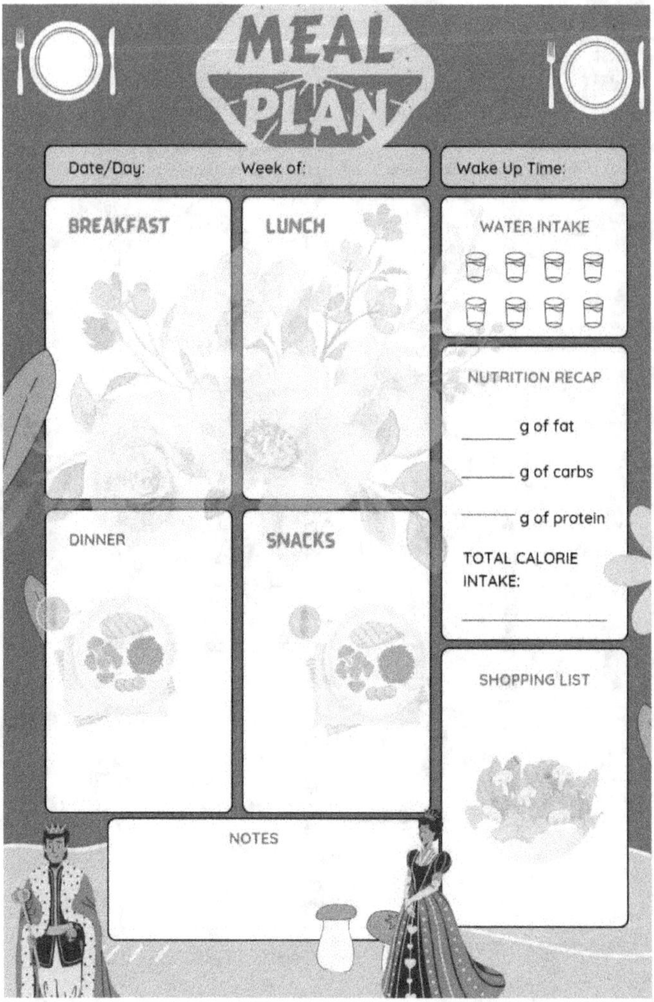

MEAL PLAN

Date/Day: Week of: Wake Up Time:

BREAKFAST

LUNCH

WATER INTAKE

NUTRITION RECAP

________ g of fat

________ g of carbs

________ g of protein

TOTAL CALORIE INTAKE:

____

DINNER

SNACKS

SHOPPING LIST

NOTES

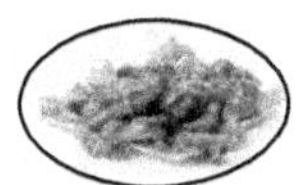 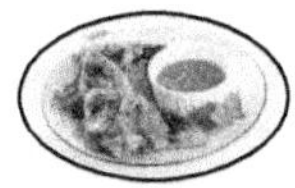 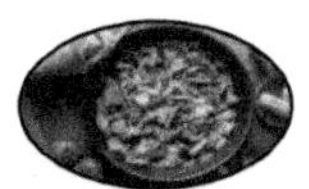

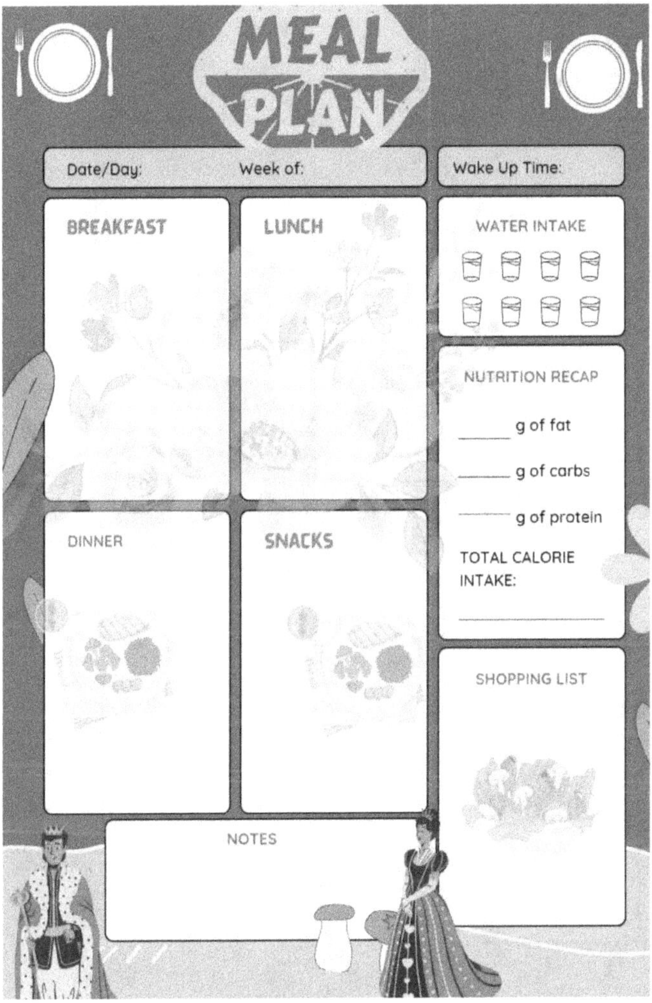

MEAL PLAN

Date/Day:	Week of:	Wake Up Time:

BREAKFAST

LUNCH

WATER INTAKE

DINNER

SNACKS

NUTRITION RECAP

________ g of fat

________ g of carbs

________ g of protein

TOTAL CALORIE INTAKE:

____

SHOPPING LIST

NOTES

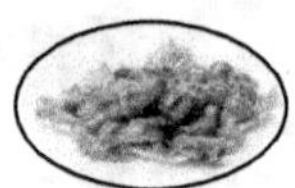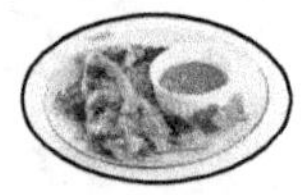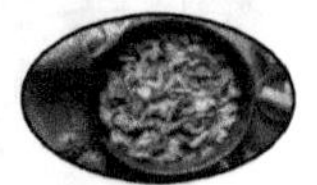

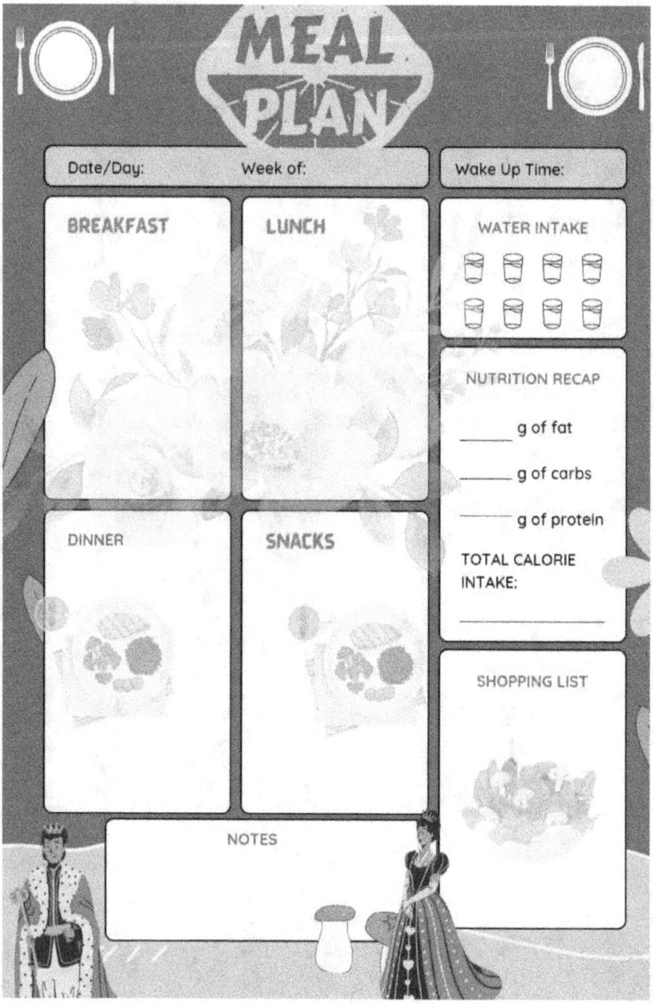

MEAL PLAN

| Date/Day: | Week of: | Wake Up Time: |

BREAKFAST

LUNCH

WATER INTAKE

NUTRITION RECAP

______ g of fat

______ g of carbs

______ g of protein

TOTAL CALORIE INTAKE:

______

DINNER

SNACKS

SHOPPING LIST

NOTES

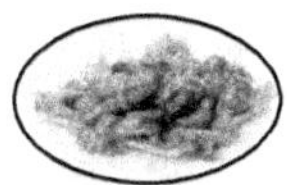 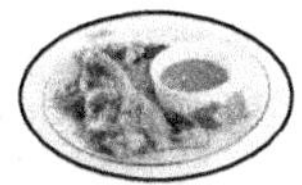 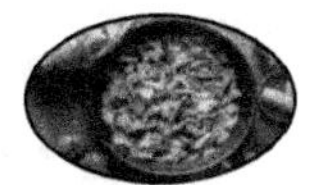

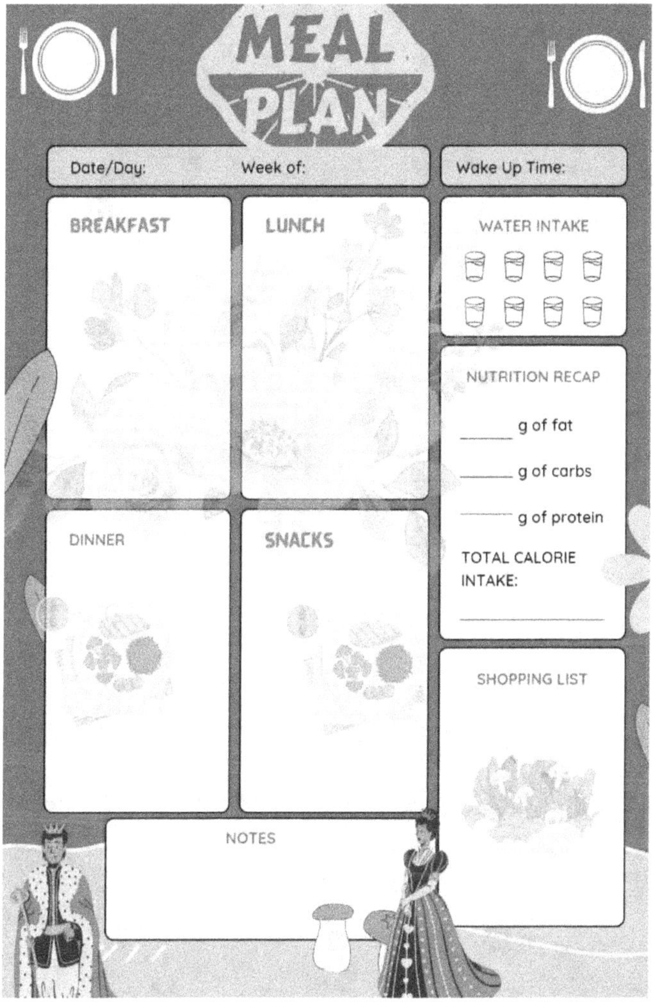

MEAL PLAN

Date/Day:	Week of:	Wake Up Time:

BREAKFAST

LUNCH

WATER INTAKE

NUTRITION RECAP

_______ g of fat

_______ g of carbs

_______ g of protein

TOTAL CALORIE INTAKE:

____

DINNER

SNACKS

SHOPPING LIST

NOTES

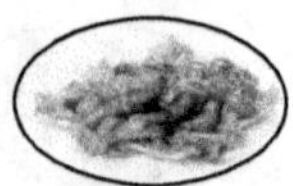
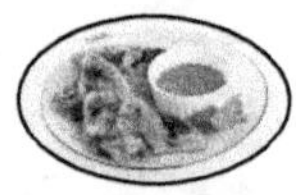
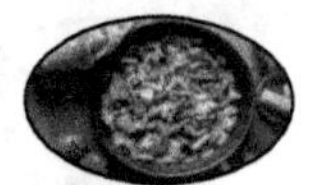

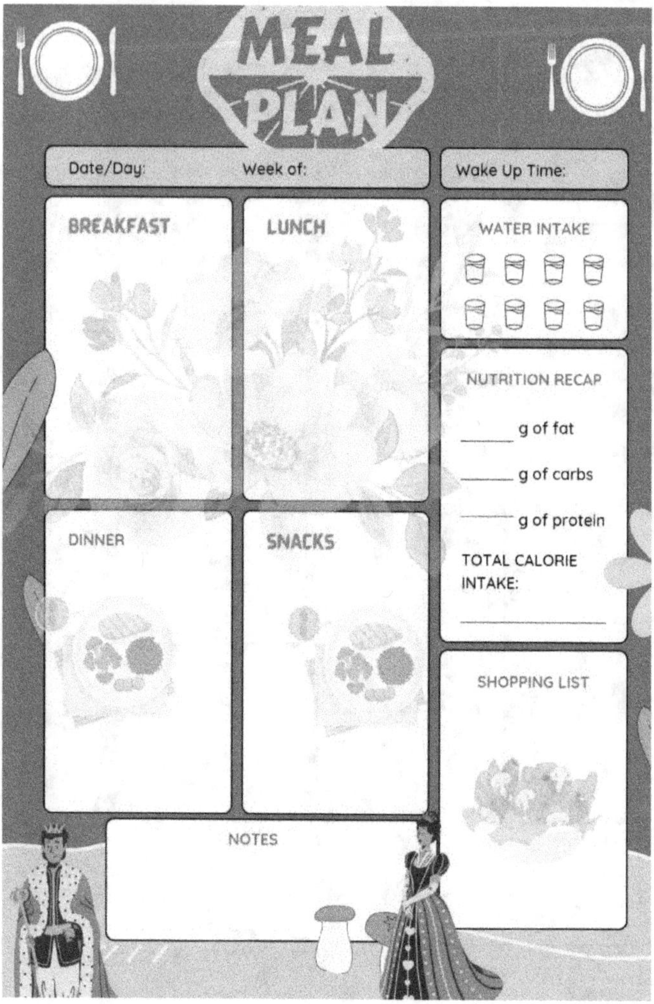

MEAL PLAN

| Date/Day: | Week of: | Wake Up Time: |

BREAKFAST

LUNCH

WATER INTAKE

NUTRITION RECAP

________ g of fat

________ g of carbs

________ g of protein

TOTAL CALORIE INTAKE:

____

DINNER

SNACKS

SHOPPING LIST

NOTES

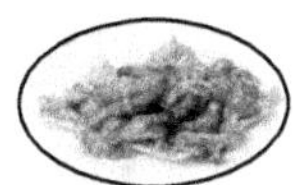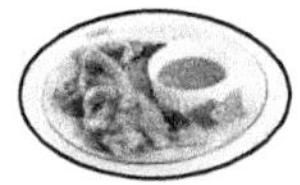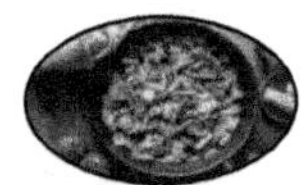

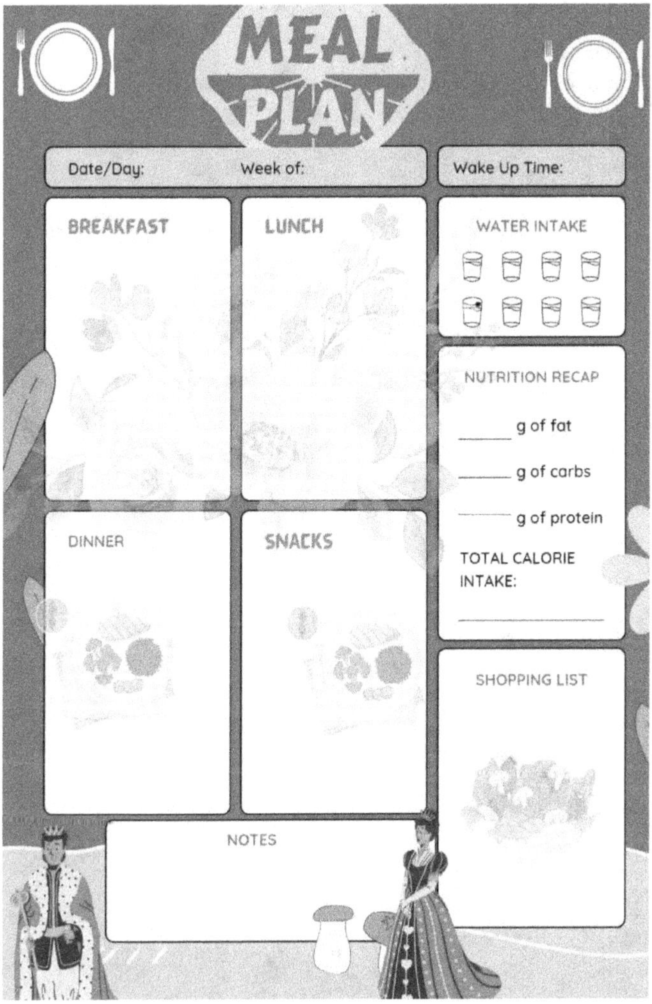

MEAL PLAN

| Date/Day: | Week of: | Wake Up Time: |

BREAKFAST

LUNCH

WATER INTAKE

NUTRITION RECAP

__________ g of fat

__________ g of carbs

__________ g of protein

TOTAL CALORIE INTAKE:

____

DINNER

SNACKS

SHOPPING LIST

NOTES

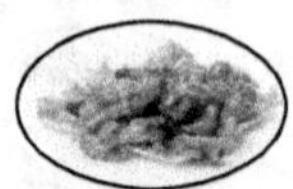 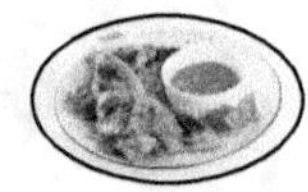 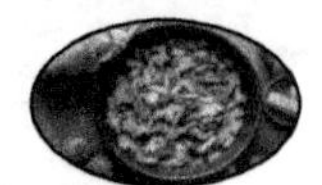

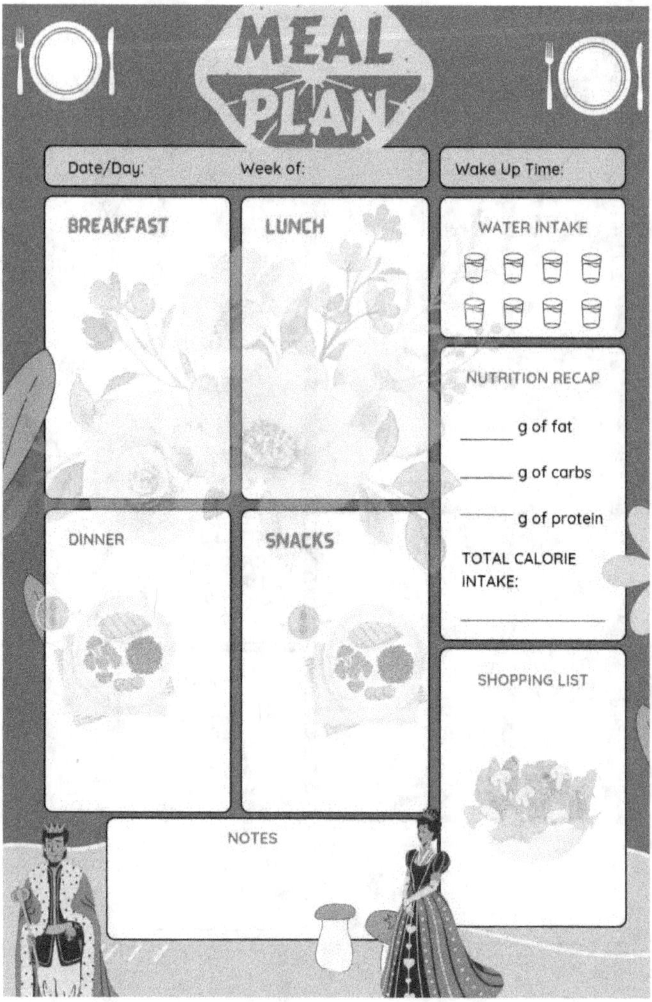

MEAL PLAN

| Date/Day: | Week of: | Wake Up Time: |

BREAKFAST

LUNCH

WATER INTAKE

NUTRITION RECAP

_______ g of fat

_______ g of carbs

_______ g of protein

TOTAL CALORIE INTAKE:

____

DINNER

SNACKS

SHOPPING LIST

NOTES

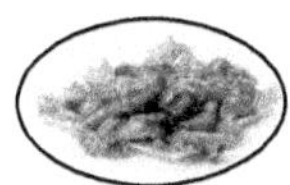 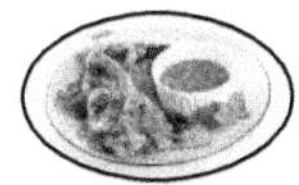 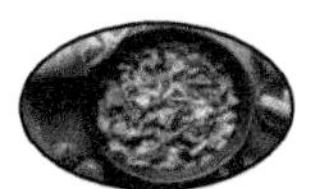

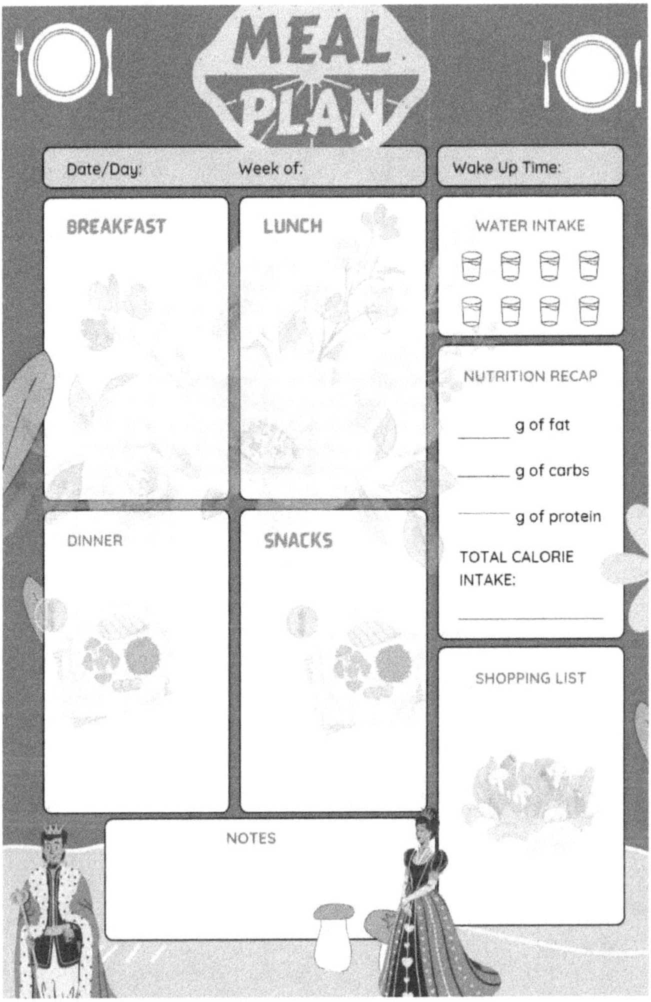

MEAL PLAN

| Date/Day: | Week of: | Wake Up Time: |

BREAKFAST

LUNCH

WATER INTAKE

NUTRITION RECAP

_______ g of fat

_______ g of carbs

_______ g of protein

TOTAL CALORIE INTAKE:

____

DINNER

SNACKS

SHOPPING LIST

NOTES